Evidence Based Medicine - what it should be, but is not

A non-systematic review
on how we ended up tyrannized

Alexander de Ru

ISBN 978-90-6299-327-7

Kugler Publications
P.O. Box 20538
1001 NM Amsterdam, The Netherlands
www.kuglerpublications.com

Kugler Publications is an imprint of SPB Academic Publishing bv, P.O. Box 20538, 1001 NM Amsterdam, The Netherlands

Table of Contents

Disclaimer

What indeed is reasonable in evidence-based medicine (EBM) is the view that certain sources of research evidence can be useful in answering certain types of questions that arise in clinical practice.[1] So, to be perfectly clear, I am not opposed to a well-balanced way of integrating research findings into medical practice.

However, the use of research evidence in practice is a good servant, but a bad master. Or, to quote Montori and Guyatt: an analogy can be made between EBM and nuclear fusion: it can be very powerful when used appropriately and dangerous when used inappropriately.[2]

Because I share the general goals and have friendly admiration for proponents of EBM, but worry about its current methods, the comments here reflect on what is actually done rather than what is proposed.[3]

Thus, 'EBM' in this book is mostly used to indicate the nihilistic approach to medicine that it has become, not the more balanced way that it, perhaps, was supposed to be.

A 'systematic review' of all criticism would probably lead to a series of books, instead of a practical and readable guide to abandoning the current narrow ways of applying EBM.

The best lines in this booklet – and actually most of its content – are not new, nor were they constructed by me. Better minds have published about this extensively; I sincerely hope the reference list will stimulate further reading. The work is not meant as form of plagiarism, but to honor the cited authors. That is why I start with the references.

References

1. Loughlin M. Reason, reality and objectivity - shared dogmas and distortions in the way both 'scientistic' and 'postmodern' commentators frame the EBM debate. J Eval Clin Pract. 2008;14:665-71. https://doi.org/10.1111/j.1365-2753.2008.01075.x

2. Montori VM, Guyatt GH. Progress in evidence based medicine. JAMA. 2008;300:1814-6. https://doi.org/10.1001/jama.300.15.1814

3. Feinstein AR, Horwitz RI. Problems in the "evidence" of "evidence-based medicine". Am J Med. 1997;103:529-35. https://doi.org/10.1016/S0002-9343(97)00244-1

4. Epstein AM. Sounding board: The outcomes movement - will it get us where we want to go. NEJM. 1990;323:266-9. https://doi.org/10.1056/NEJM199007263230410

5. Charlton BG, Miles A. The rise and fall of EBM. Q J Med. 1998;91:371-4. https://doi.org/10.1093/qjmed/91.5.371

6. Upshur R. Making the grade; assuring trustworthiness in evidence. Perspect Biol Med. 2009;52:264-75. https://doi.org/10.1353/pbm.0.0079

7. Miller CG. Re: distinguishing opinion from evidence in guidelines. Rapid response to BMJ. 2019;366:l4606. https://doi.org/10.1136/bmj.l4606

8. Anderson T, Schum D, Twining W. Analysis of Evidence. 3rd printing. Cambridge: Cambridge University Press; 2009.

9. Upshur REG, Colak E. Argumentation and Evidence. Theor Med. 2003;24:283-99. https://doi.org/10.1023/A:1026006801902

10. Jenicek M. Evidence-based medicine. Fifteen years later. Golem the good, the bad, and the ugly in need of revision. Med Sci Monit. 2006;12:RA241-51.

11. Jenicek M. The hard art of soft science: evidence-based medicine, reasoned medicine or both. J Eval Clin Pract. 2006;12:410-9. https://doi.org/10.1111/j.1365-2753.2006.00718.x

12. Pellegrino ED. The ethical use of evidence in biomedicine. Eval Health Prof. 1999;22:33-43. https://doi.org/10.1177/01632789922034158

13. Shahar E. A Popperian perspective of the term 'evidence-based medicine'. J Eval Clin Pract. 1997;3:109-16. https://doi.org/10.1046/j.1365-2753.1997.00092.x

14. Mills ES. QuickLesson 8: What Constitutes Proof? Evidence Explained: Historical Analysis, Citation & Source Usage. [Internet]. [cited 2023 Dec 30]. Available from: https://www.evidenceexplained.com/content/quicklesson-8-what-constitutes-proof.

15. Anderson AA. Assessing statistical results: magnitude, precision and model uncertainty. Am Stat. 2019;73(S1):118-21. https://doi.org/10.1080/00031305.2018.1537889

16. Tanenbaum SJ. Evidence and expertise: the challenge of the outcomes movement to medical professionalism. Acad Med. 1999;74:757-63. https://doi.org/10.1097/00001888-199907000-00008

17. Engebretsen E, Vollestad NK, Wahl AK, Robinson HS, Heggen K. Unpacking the process of interpretation in evidence-based decision making. J Eval Clin Pract. 2015;21:529-31. https://doi.org/10.1111/jep.12362

18. Tanenbaum SJ. Sounding Board: what physicians know. NEJM. 1993;329:1268-70. https://doi.org/10.1056/NEJM199310213291713

19. Guyatt G, Cairns J, Churchill D. Evidence-Based Medicine - a new approach to teaching the practice of medicine. JAMA. 1992;268:2420-5. https://doi.org/10.1001/jama.1992.03490170092032

20. Charlton BG. Jacob Bronowski's principle of tolerance. Med Hypotheses. 2007;70:215-7. https://doi.org/10.1016/j.mehy.2007.07.028

21. Tonelli MR. Integrating evidence into clinical practice: an alternative to evidence-based approaches. J Eval Clin Pract. 2006;12:248-56. https://doi.org/10.1111/j.1365-2753.2004.00551.x

22. McShane BB, Gal B, Gelman A, Robert C, Tackett JL. Abandon statistical significance. Am Stat. 2019;73:235-45. https://doi.org/10.1080/00 031305.2018.1527253

23. Evans JG. Evidence-based and evidence-biased medicine? Age Ageing. 1995;24:461-3. https://doi.org/10.1093/ageing/24.6.461

24. Miles A, Polychronis A, Grey JE. The evidence-based health care debate - 2006. Where are we now? J Eval Clin Pract. 2006;12:239-47. https://doi.org/10.1111/j.1365-2753.2006.00709.x

25. Hunter DJ. Rationing and evidence-based medicine. J Eval Clin Pract. 1996;2:5-8. https://doi.org/10.1111/j.1365-2753.1996.tb00023.x

26. Charlton BG. Restoring the balance: evidence-based medicine put in its place. J Eval Clin Pract. 1997;3:87-98. https://doi.org/10.1046/j.1365-2753.1997.00097.x

27. Horwitz RI. The dark side of evidence-based medicine. Cleve Clin J Med. 1996;63:320-3. https://doi.org/10.3949/ccjm.63.6.320

28. Cochrane A. Effectiveness and efficiency. In: random reflections on health services. The Nuffield Provincial Hospital Trust ed. [Internet]. [cited 1972 Jun 1, last accessed 2021 Feb 17]. Available from: http://www.nuffieldtrust.org.uk/research/effectiveness-and-efficiency-random-reflections-on-health-services.

29. Steel EA, Liermann M, Guttorp P. Beyond calculations: a course in statistical thinking. Am Stat. 2019;73(S1):392-401. https://doi.org/10.1080/00031305.2018.1505657

30. Smulders Y. Evidence based: to be or not to be? Ned J Med. 2011;69(2):53-4.

31. Hofmeijer J. Evidence-based knowledge: the neglected role of expert opinion. J Eval Clin Pract. 2014;20:803-8. https://doi.org/10.1111/jep.12267

32. Haynes RB. What kind of evidence is it that Evidence-Based Medicine advocates want health care providers and consumers to pay attention to? BMC Health Serv Res. 2002;2:3. https://doi.org/10.1186/1472-6963-2-3

33. Porta M. Is there life after evidence-based medicine? J Eval Clin Pract. 2003;10:147-52. https://doi.org/10.1111/j.1365-2753.2003.00473.x

34. Spodich DH. "Evidence-based medicine": terminologic lapse or terminologic arrogance? Am J Cardiol. 1996;78:608-9. https://doi.org/10.1016/S0002-9149(96)90531-7

35. Upshur REG, Tracy CS. Legitimacy, authority, and hierarchy: critical challenges for evidence-based medicine. Brief Treat Crisis Interv. 2004;4:197-204. https://doi.org/10.1093/brief-treatment/mhh018

36. Steinberg EP, Luce BR. Evidence based? Caveat emptor. Health Aff (Millwood). 2005;24:80-92. https://doi.org/10.1377/hlthaff.24.1.80

37. Djulbegovic B, Guyatt GH, Ashcroft RE. Epistemologic inquiries in evidence-based medicine. Cancer Control. 2009;16:158-68. https://doi.org/10.1177/107327480901600208

38. Goodman S. Why is getting rid of p-values so hard? Musings on science and statistics. Am Stat. 2019;73(S1):26-30. https://doi.org/10.1080/00031305.2018.1558111

39. Tonelli MR. The philosophical limits of evidence-based medicine. Acad Med. 1998;73:1234-40. https://doi.org/10.1097/00001888-199812000-00011

40. Henry SG, Zaner RM, Dittus RS. Viewpoint: moving beyond evidence-based medicine. Acad Med. 2007;82:292-7. https://doi.org/10.1097/ACM.0b013e3180307f6d

41. Norman GR. Examining the assumptions of evidence-based medicine. J Eval Clin Pract. 1999;5:139-47. https://doi.org/10.1046/j.1365-2753.1999.00197.x

42. Sackett DL, Rosenberg WM, Gray JA, Haynes RB, Richardson WS. Evidence based medicine: what it is and what it isn't. BMJ. 1996;312(7023):71-2. https://doi.org/10.1136/bmj.312.7023.71

43. Loughlin M. The basis of medical knowledge: judgement, objectivity and the history of ideas. J Eval Clin Pract. 2009;15:935-40. https://doi.org/10.1111/j.1365-2753.2009.01318.x

44. Tonelli MR. In defense of expert opinion. Acad Med. 1999;74:1187-92. https://doi.org/10.1097/00001888-199911000-00010

45. Van Baalen S, Boon M. An epistemological shift: from evidence-based medicine to epistemological responsibility. J Eval Clin Pract. 2015;21:433-9. https://doi.org/10.1111/jep.12282

46. Miles A, Bentley P, Polychronis A, Grey J. Evidence-based medicine: why all the fuss? This is why. J Eval Clin Pract. 1997;3:83-6. https://doi.org/10.1046/j.1365-2753.1997.00103.x

47. Karanicolas PJ, Kunz R, Guyatt GH. Evidence-based medicine has a sound scientific base. Chest. 2008;133:1067-71. https://doi.org/10.1378/chest.08-0068

48. Hatala R, Guyatt G. Evaluating the teaching of evidence-based medicine. JAMA. 2002;288:1110-1. https://doi.org/10.1001/jama.288.9.1110

49. Greenhalgh TF. Of lamp posts, keys, and fabled drunkards; a perspectival tale of 4 guidelines. J Eval Clin Pract. 2018;24:1132-8. https://doi.org/10.1111/jep.12925

50. Horton R. The interpretive turn. Lancet. 1995;346:3. https://doi.org/10.1016/S0140-6736(95)92644-5

51. Charlton BG. Public Health versus Personal Health. Public Health. 1993;107:397-9. https://doi.org/10.1016/S0033-3506(05)80163-5

52. Clinicians for the Restoration of Autonomous Practice (CRAP) Writing Group. EBM: un-masking the ugly truth. BMJ. 2002 Dec 21;325(7378):1496-8. https://doi.org/10.1136/bmj.325.7378.1496

53. Rawlins M. De testimonio: on the evidence for decisions about the use of therapeutic interventions. Lancet. 2008;372(9656):2152-1. https://doi.org/10.1016/S0140-6736(08)61930-3

54. Sackett DL, Wennberg JE. Choosing the best research design for each question. It's time to stop squabbling over the "best" methods. BMJ. 1997;315:1636. https://doi.org/10.1136/bmj.315.7123.1636

55. Hadorn DC, Baker D, Hodges JS, Hicks N. Rating the quality of evidence for clinical practice guidelines. J Clin Epidemiol. 1996;49:749-54. https://doi.org/10.1016/0895-4356(96)00019-4

56. Elstein AS. Thinking about diagnostic thinking: a 30-year perspective. Adv Health Sci Educ. 2009;14:7-18. https://doi.org/10.1007/s10459-009-9184-0

57. Maier T. Evidence-based psychiatry: understanding the limitations of a method. J Eval Clin Pract. 2006;12:325-9. https://doi.org/10.1111/j.1365-2753.2006.00604.x

58. Gill P, Dowell AC, Neal RD, Smith N, Heywood P, Wilson AE. Evidence based general practice: a retrospective study of interventions in one training practice. BMJ. 1996;312:819-21. https://doi.org/10.1136/bmj.312.7034.819

59. Hill AB. The environment and disease: association or causation? Proc Royal Soc Med. 1965;58:295-300. https://doi.org/10.1177/003591576505800503

60. Charlton BG. Philosophy of medicine: alternative or scientific. J R Soc Med. 1992;85:436-8. https://doi.org/10.1177/014107689208500802

61. Chalmers I, Sackett D, Silagy C. In: Maynard A, Chalmers I. Non-random reflections on health services research. 1999. [Internet]. [cited 1997 Mar 1, last accessed 2021 Feb 17]. Available from: http://www.nuffieldtrust.org.uk/research/non-random-reflections-on-health-services-research.

62. Sleigh JW. Logical limits of randomized controlled trials. J Eval Clin Pract. 1997;3:145-8. https://doi.org/10.1046/j.1365-2753.1997.00068.x

63. Amrhein V, Trafimow D, Greenland S. Inferential statistics as descriptive statistics: there is no replication crisis if we don't expect replication. Am Stat. 2019;73(S1):262-70. https://doi.org/10.1080/00031305.2018.1543137

64. Jenicek M. Towards evidence-based critical thinking medicine? Uses of best evidence in flawless argumentations. Med Sci Monit. 2006;12:RA149-53.

65. Canadian Task Force on the periodic Health Examination. The periodic health examination. CMAJ. 1979;121:1193-206.

66. De Ru JA. Epidemiology, the cherry on the cake. Eur Arch Otorhinolaryngol. 2022;279:1645-8. https://doi.org/10.1007/s00405-021-07179-5

EBM; what it should be, but is not

A non-systematic review on how we ended up tyrannized

> *"When I use a word,"* Humpty Dumpty said, in a rather scornful tone, *"it means just what I choose it to mean – neither more nor less."* – Lewis Carroll

Nowadays, EBM is apparently being practiced and taught as looking especially at randomized controlled trials (RCTs) and meta-analysis.[3] Medical students are brainwashed into dogmatic, narrow ways of applying EBM. Medical knowledge and sound clinical judgement, have become inferior to literature assessment.

When asked about EBM, it seems that many young colleagues had quite an extensive training in critical appraisal of studies, however, they had not been presented with any of the opposing views.

In 1990, Epstein warned already that the danger we faced was that we would undermine a healthy evolution and allow revolutionary zeal to lead us to carry a good thing too fast and too far.[4] I fear that this has come true.

Because of the guidelines I read and have to comply to, the students and residents I talk to, the discussions I have while collaborating with epidemiologists in research, and the reviewers' comments I obtained during the last decade, I thought it necessary to show the other side of the medal again, summarized in this booklet with the many quotes of predecessors.

As Charlton and Miles already stated in 1998, the time is ripe for the 'evidence-based' mantra to be silenced and dissenting voices to be heard. If EBM does not fall spontaneously, it may need to be pushed.[5]

Conclusions

1. Only a very small amount of all available evidence is currently used as 'evidence' in EBM.

2. Many self-described EBM practitioners interpret 'evidence' in a dogmatic, narrow view as only deriving from study results; especially systematic reviews of RCTs are accepted as the gold standard.

3. Medicine cannot function without clinical expertise and expert opinion – these are a sine qua non even in all of the steps proposed in EBM; they should not have been devalued.

4. EBM is not a new paradigm and should not have been promoted as such.

5. The interests between public health care and individual care for a patient might differ.

6. EBM in patient care is not what it should be.

1. What is evidence?

"The chief danger to philosophy is narrowness in the selection of evidence. This narrowness arises from the idiosyncrasies and timidities of particular authors, of particular social groups, of particular schools of thought, of particular epochs in the history of civilization. The evidence relied upon is arbitrarily biased by the temperaments of individuals, by provincialities of groups and by the limitation of schemes of thought." –
Alfred North Whitehead[6]

Evidence is information; it can be any information; it can be true or false; it must be relevant. Relevance is its tendency to support or undermine a disputed proposition; if it is not disputed no evidence supporting is needed. Undermining evidence makes the proposition disputed.[7]

The Federal rules of Evidence in the United States provide a useful definition: 'relevant evidence' means evidence having any tendency to make the existence of any fact that is of consequence to the determination of the action more probable or less probable than it would be without the evidence.[8]

These definitions intertwined in medicine would have been enough to create EBM. Alas, medicine and health care are not traditionally associated with concerns for argumentation and its evaluation. Medical professionals seem to ignore human knowledge external to medicine; medical literature concerning evidence is consequently populated by metaphorical re-invented square and triangular wheels.[7]

The advent of EBM has raised issues relating to epistemology, philosophy of science, and informal logic.[9] Within the general scope of evidence, as seen by philosophers/critical thinkers, falls not only a demonstration of causality, but also intuition, personal experience, testimonials, appeals to authorities, personal observations, case examples, research studies, and analogies.[10] Such an enlarged spectrum of evidence calls for a more refined view of evidence in medicine.

A viable concept of evidence for practical use in medicine might be formulated as any data or information, whether solid or weak, obtained through experience, observational research or experimental work. These data or information must be relevant and convincing to some degree either to the understanding of the problem (case) or to the clinical decisions (diagnostic, therapeutic, or care-oriented) made about the case.[11]

Evidence does not mean certainty. The evidentiary basis for belief may not be necessarily true. Evidence is not automatically correct, complete, satisfactory and useful.[11] It must first be evaluated, graded and based on its own merit.[11] Particular claims can be confirmed by given evidence to various degrees.

Evidence can be misleading. How do we know whether what is provided (*i.e.*, what is logically correct) is also true (*i.e.*, congruent with reality)?[12] There are assertions which are held to be true by some people, by many people, or by practically everyone, and might be false, regardless of how many believers line up to support them.[13]

The evidence in studies is stronger when the effect is large, cannot be explained by bias and chance, and when it is replicated in other studies. The totality of evidence often has greater probative value than the sum of the parts. Consequently, EBM must encourage doctors to consider all potentially relevant kinds of medical knowledge in each case.

The strength of any piece of evidence rests with its power to convince that our assertions square with some reality external to our minds.[12] As with any construction project, results are only as good as the materials and the labor we invest.[14] Evidence can be compatible with more than one explanation and there is no logical basis to derive the truthfulness or falseness of any statement. A statement is verifiable if it can be supported by direct observation or if we can use it to derive statements that are themselves directly verifiable and cannot be derived without it. According to Popper, a scientific hypothesis can never be proven; it can only be falsified or rejected. If after rigorous testing the hypothesis is not refuted, it remains corroborated.

Proof is a body of evidence. What constitutes sufficient evidence?[12]

We may also ask ourselves which standard of proof is required for each and every decision we make. Beyond reasonable doubt, clear and convincing, or simply that a possibility exists (the preponderance of the evidence/the balance of the probabilities)?[8]

We do not 'prove' a point by discovering a record that asserts something. That assertion could be wrong. If so, any further work we do on the basis of that misinformation will likely be wrong or irrelevant.[14]

Achieving 'proof' is a process in which we assemble evidence, test it, refine it, and reinforce it until that body of evidence is solid enough to withstand contradictions and counterclaims.[14] Accumulated evidence from multiple studies may eventually satisfy a 'burden of proof', but individual studies are rarely definitive.[15]

Even if empirical experience is consistent and we are lucky enough to reach unanimous agreement about the interpretation of cumulative empirical experience, it is still unclear at what point of time we have gathered 'enough' evidence to justify an action.[13] What is the logical answer to the question of how many times a successful trial should be replicated to allow for a claim of proof? Does one mega-trial provide the evidence whereas three small trials do not, or vice versa?[13] Does a doctor who adopts some therapy after its first successful test practice EBM, whereas a doctor who postpones his decision until that therapy has withstood five tests practices *non-evidence based medicine*, or vice versa?[13]

2. Uncertainty

Uncertainty is inherent in medical practice because patients present individual and complex medical circumstances. Medical professionals do not pursue certainty, but wisdom under conditions of uncertainty.[16]

In an act of interpretation, not application, physicians make clinical sense of a case, rather than placing it in a general category of cases. As interpreters, physicians draw on all their knowledge, but even the integration of all relevant findings creates an incomplete picture. There is always more to the issue than the doctor can possibly uncover through his investigation.[17] No physician can know a patient in his or her entirety or be certain what inferences to draw from aggregate studies.[18] The patient in all his or her particularity takes precedence over aggregations, however informative.[16]

Clinical evidence is not perfect: patients may not tell entirely accurate histories, physical findings and laboratory tests do not perfectly distinguish between diseased and disease-free populations, sensitivity and specificity are typically <1. For example, the morphologic data routinely provided by pathologists and radiologists is readily accepted, despite the inconsistencies and biases revealed by interobserver variability.[3] So, what professionals know is inherently and irreparably uncertain;[16] that is the ineradicable uncertainty at the core of the medical enterprise. We must know how to recognize uncertainty and its degrees.[12]

In this sense, clinical medicine is essentially fallible; a limitation that EBM is powerless to remedy. Even according to the EBM working group (EBMWG), clinicians must be ready to accept and live with uncertainty and to acknowledge that management decisions are often made in the face of relative ignorance of their true impact.[19]

But professionalism accepts uncertainty and the fallibility that follows from it.[16] Professionals gather necessarily incomplete information that may include, among other things, outcomes research (OR), and arrive at an always imperfect understanding that can nevertheless be judged against standards of perceptiveness, coherence, etc.[16] This clinical sense-making continuously revises itself and allows for accountable action on the patient's behalf at any time.[16] You have to tell the truth the way you see it. And yet you have to be tolerant of the fact that neither you nor the person you are arguing with is going to get it right.[20]

Clinical decision-making is a personal and prudential undertaking and therefore clinicians may arrive at different conclusions in similar cases.[21]

The inherent fallibility of medical knowledge indicates that the type of reasoning employed by physicians is more provisional in nature, pragmatic in orientation and probabilistic in its expression.[9] Judgements and decisions in clinical medicine rest more on plausibility than certainty, that is, what seems to be true or appropriate in a given set of circumstances.[9] What is plausible and reasonable to do in a clinical encounter is determined by the context of that clinical encounter, not by the existence of research evidence.[9] Plausible inferences intend to provide a reasonable guide for sustaining a belief or justifying an action, but may in fact turn out to be erroneous, and in need of revision.[9] This is consistent with the nature of medical evidence.

The acceptance of variability, however, runs counter to one of the stated benefits of EBM, the limiting of practice variability.[21] The claim by EBM proponents seems to be the untenable one that strong or high-quality evidence with magnitude of effect stated in some probability statement, is sufficient to secure 'certainty'.[6] How the determination of sufficient robustness is determined is unclear.[6] It seems to entail some form of consensus or convention around acceptable bounds of uncertainty, largely without any input or discussion on how these bounds are set.[6] A form of statistical alchemy that falsely promises to transmute randomness into certainty.[22]

It obscures and directs attention away from the inherent uncertainties present in even the best evidence.[6]

Epidemiological assumptions claiming 'evidence' at points it does not exist, or that consist of just a small part of the available evidence, are very much misleading for the ignorant. It leads clinicians to search for evidence in systematic reviews of trials only, whereas the major part of the evidence will be found in the remaining literature, in logic, pathophysiologic rationale, clinical experience, etc., together. That is like the search of the drunkard for his car keys under the lamp post; not because he dropped them there, but because it was where the light shone.[23]

EBM's continuing attraction appears to be based on some clinicians' need for certainty in the inherently uncertain world of clinical practice.[24] This constitutes 'uncertainty laundering'; and it risks synthesizing a 'false certainty', far more liable to result in suboptimal care at the least and error and injury at the worst, than the exercise of what has been pejoratively described as 'traditional' clinical medicine with its well-established emphasis on caution, experience and consensus.[24]

The search for objectivity, it would seem, has no place for judgement and yet judgement is critical in medicine when its practitioners are faced with the uniqueness of each individual patient as well as with the uncertainties inherent in medicine.[25]

In the principle of tolerance, Bronowski stated that "all information is imperfect" and that "our ability to work and act in the real world depends on our accepting a tolerance in our recognition and language".[20] The principle of tolerance is the judgement that two instances are sufficiently similar that we can treat them as the same for present purposes.[20] Too much tolerance and science becomes unreliable because you are misled by random variation; too little tolerance and you lose valuable information.[20] The too-credulous scientist may be spinning a story based on foundations of sand; but the ultra-sceptic will block progress by knocking-down every potential advance.[20] The scientific process depends on an understanding that the best scientific result in the world is not *right*, but that the best experiment in the world is surrounded by an area of tolerance.[20] There are thus two pressures in science. One is to strive for ever-lower levels of tolerance and to seek ever-greater levels of precision in measurement. The other is to accept a reasonable, attainable level of tolerance so that work can proceed now.[20]

3. Epidemiology

Initially, EBM grew as a bottom-up approach to continuing medical education under the name of clinical epidemiology (CE).[5] It was inaugurated and led by epidemiologists. Hence, epidemiology was not an 'emphasis' or a 'focus' of EBM; rather, EBM was an extension and expansion of clinical epidemiology into the domain of clinical practice. The outcomes movement (OM), with lots of insurance data and enhanced computer capacity, sought to make it the gold standard.

EBM intended to instill within clinicians the ability to independently and critically read the biomedical research literature. In other words, it was a research literacy movement. In retrospect, the positive effects of this epidemiological emphasis were exaggerated and its problems and insufficiencies were never properly addressed — nonetheless CE was widely regarded as a refreshing approach that blew away cobwebs and let in some light.[5] In particular, CE mobilized the enthusiasm of people to come to grips with interpreting clinical data for themselves for use in their own clinical practice.[5]

But the advocates of CE were ambitious of influence, and grew impatient. A significant change came when the name 'Evidence-Based Medicine' or EBM was coined in 1992.[5,19] Since adopting its new title, the technical toolkit once termed 'clinical epidemiology' has undergone a neoplastic growth to form that *total system* called EBM.[26] The protagonists of CE have moved towards establishing an interlocking set of mutually supportive proposals for reorganizing the whole of medical practice – medical education, the daily activities of clinical medicine, economic decisions, health policy, rationing and management; all these (and more) to be integrated and brought under the evidence-based (EB) banner.[26]

CE was based upon emphasizing the potential of epidemiological information for guiding clinical practice. But one needs to remember that epidemiology is a set of statistical methods and investigational techniques for summarizing and analyzing health states in populations.[26] Epidemiology is more like a toolkit for clinical scientists – a method for measuring health variables with high precision through sampling large populations.[26] But for a toolkit to be valuable, it must be used for the right job by people with the necessary skills: measurements are worthless unless we know what to measure and why.[26]

Epidemiology is a technical not a scientific discipline. But like other techniques, it has the capacity to distort science, to frame questions and drive investigation by that which is technically most feasible.[26] Indeed, EBM is characterized – if anything – by its denigration of science, and by pointing out the potential for knowledge derived from the basic medical sciences (such as physiology, biochemistry and pharmacology) to be misleading when applied to clinical circumstances.[26] Although I concur with the fact that laboratory science must be interpreted carefully when applied to the vastly more complicated and uncontrolled circumstances of human disease; careful interpretation is something different from de-emphasizing. EBM gives primacy to the application of probabilistic research. The evidence in EBM, then, is that derived from researchers' statistical analysis across individuals – evidence of likelihood in the aggregate.[16] Consequently, the 'input' used by EBM is not necessarily valid knowledge at all – it may simply be a statistical summary of an aggregation of data; a measurement, the validity of which is unknown.[26] A quantified association between variables may not represent coherent biological entities or their interaction.[26] The validity of EBM data is determined by there being sufficient scientific knowledge of the circumstances under which the data were gathered to enable one to argue legitimately that the variables measured represent real biological entities, and that the association between them represents a causal process.[26]

It is not merely a question of EBM results being of limited relevance – they may be of no relevance, and only prior relevant knowledge can tell us whether this is so.[26] In the absence of contextual information, EBM is only a set of methods for gathering and interpreting data – a flow chart combining information technology with biostatistics and a set of arbitrary rules of inference.[26] Just because a model is statistical does not mean it is more valid than a non-quantitative model – it merely means that the model is more exactly quantified, and hence more precisely predictive and more readily testable.[26] Still, statistics should be the servants of science: they cannot be allowed to dictate science.

Relying excessively on epidemiological evidence is a danger that we are insufficiently aware of. Alas, from an EBM point of view only experimental evidence, especially results from randomized controlled trials and meta-analyses of trial results, count as strong evidence.[17]

4. Outcomes Movement

The OM dates from the early 1970s, when rising healthcare costs and new research on health care utilization cast serious doubt on the existing knowledge base for medical practice.[16] Origins of the OM were: (1) need for cost containment; (2) competition between insurers; and (3) geographical differences in the use of various medical procedures.[4]

The OM accepts as axiomatic that a substantial portion of health care expenditure in the US was wasted on unproven or ineffective tests and treatment.[18,27] The unspoken conviction of the OM was that impersonal knowledge of the probability of an event is the principal precondition for effective clinical medicine and superior to the more traditional physician learning-by-experience and the pathophysiologic reasoning.[27]

In patient care, evidence from clinical research should supplant intuition, clinical experience and physiologic rationale.[18,27] This was in line with the work of Archibald Cochrane, one of the great epidemiologists from the last century.[28]

The OM was described as the obvious response to findings of unexplained and ostensibly wasteful variation in physicians' practice patterns.[18] This variation was thought to result from uncertainty.[18] The goals of the OM were to bring order and predictability to the American health care system and to bring physician accountability to patients and providers of health care. Implementation would make more efficient use of the country's resources. 'Small area variation studies' raised the troubling question of why physicians in different communities attempted to solve the same medical problem in different ways.[16] Variations research was widely interpreted to mean that physicians were uncertain about the values of alternative treatments and that their actions were consequently influenced by clinically extraneous factors such as tradition or convenience.[16] This led to an attempt to reduce the uncertainty by research on effectiveness. However: one might ask if variations mean unnecessary costs in high-use areas or less than optimal care in low-use areas?[4] Virtually all studies on appropriateness so far and much of the attendant dialogue have focused on patients who undergo unnecessary procedures rather than on patients who do not receive appropriate care. I suspect that a reduction in the cost of care is high on the silent agenda.[4] As a result, administrative efforts are more likely to be focused on decreasing inappropriate care than on increasing access to beneficial procedures.[4]

Furthermore, by chance alone, we nearly always see the highest and lowest disease rates in the smallest counties.[29] This might explain differences in the number of surgeries performed and other variations as well.

Proponents of the new emphasis on measuring the outcomes of medical practice predicted myriad social benefits, including better information for both physicians and patients, improved guidelines for medical practice, and wiser decisions by purchasers of health care. These include increased understanding of the effectiveness of different interventions, the use of this information for better decision making by physicians and patients, and the development of standards to guide physicians and aid third-party payers in optimizing the use of resources.

The Health Care Financing Administration and the Agency for Health Care Policy and Research (AHCPR), launched a program directed at gauging the effectiveness of medical interventions and developing guidelines for medical practice through the assessment of patient outcomes.[4] The AHCPR would encourage physicians and other healthcare providers to change their practice patterns presumably by persuading them to use OR findings to make clinical decisions.[16]

Specifically, the OM promised to make health care more effective by requiring physicians to act on information from statistical analyses of large data bases.[18] It is perhaps a linguistic confusion, but many people have grabbed on to the idea that statistical significance is in some way related to proof of causation.[26] This is a profound error, although a common one; statistical proof has, in logical terms, nothing at all to do with causation.[26]

The OM sets the unrealistic goal of creating important certainties for practitioners. The movement thereby misrepresented the terms of the clinical encounter and inadvertently undermined confidence in the physician's ability to act wisely in the face of inevitable uncertainty. The OM challenges professionalism by disputing what and how physicians know, and especially by marginalizing what one physician can know about one patient.[16] It values statistical probabilism above all other forms of medical knowledge, while at the same time devaluing most of what goes by the name clinical judgement.[16] The OM maintains that measurements across patients surpasses the physician's knowledge of a single patient. Such probabilistic research can be seen, then, as scientific grounds for lay management of physician behavior.[16]

The movement's knowledge hierarchy disempowers practicing physicians relative to probabilistic researchers, and it equates clinical skill with applied science.[16] The OM radically circumscribes the usefulness of physician practice to medical knowledge.[16] According to the OM, a physician's experience contributes little to, and may actually subvert, medical knowledge.[16]

But, how will the physician incorporate outcomes data when making the multiple consecutive decisions that characterize patient care?[18] Pause at each juncture to determine whether data on effectiveness exist?[18] How much clinical intelligence will be lost in such a rigid system?[18]

The OM requires knowledge to be objective and to create certainty; professionals use objective and subjective knowledge and act in spite of uncertainty.[16] The OM joins knowledge and practice through application while professionalism does it through interpretation. Whereas the OM promotes following rules, professionals think intuitively and in context.[16] By mistaking a part of medical knowledge for the whole, the OM devalues clinical expertise and ultimately clinical medicine itself.[18]

Ultimately, the movement justifies, and even advocates, molding physicians' behavior to match as closely as possible a 'best' form of medical practice, by hortatory, economic, or regulatory means.[18]

OR is increasingly used to justify policies regulating practice, including consensus statements, practice guidelines, and practice protocols, which are offered in turn as standards for third-party reimbursement and malpractice litigation.[4] This happens in care institutions, such as hospitals, as well as in political and financial institutions, where the narrow definition of EBM is abused to regulate care and its associated costs.[30]

To conclude, OM was intended to serve Public Health Care and not for individual doctors and patients. The OM was motivated by a desire for certainty, although this can be only certainty of a likelihood.[16]

5. EBM

The concept EBM first appeared in medical literature in 1991, but it drew wider attention following an article in *JAMA* a year later.[19] According to that paper, the former paradigm did not make much use of the literature; reading the introduction and discussion section of a paper could be considered an appropriate way of gaining the relevant information from a current journal.[19] That, however, seems to be a rather simplified and exaggerated assumption. We must keep in mind that for example the *Lancet* already existed 150 years before publication of said article, and that centuries before that paper was presented, doctors were publishing books and theses already as a form of education or scientific progress; so they were making use of the literature in all its facets.

The 1992 paper challenged the preeminence of physiological (causal-inductive) reasoning in medicine.

EBM claimed to be founded on the scientific method, where new knowledge results from experimental evidence, subjected to specific principles of reasoning.[31] In EBM, the revision of valid evidence is mainly driven by the aim to deprive it from subjectivity.[31] It was proposed as an empirically adequate standard of reasonable practice and it was intended to be a means of increasing certainty at the expense of intuition, unsystematic clinical experience with patients, and pathological-physiological rationale.[10] The factors driving interest in EB decision-making were essentially the same factors that earlier drove interest in OR. A lack of reliable evidence was supposed to be the chief source of a well-documented variation in the practice of medicine. Using 'the best' available research evidence would place clinical decision-making on a more objective basis.[9] Furthermore, the use of research evidence in practice would reduce unnecessary variations in practice, lessen arbitrariness in the use of prescription medication and diagnostic testing, and eliminate the influence of values in decision making.[9]

A fundamental assumption of EBM is that practitioners whose practice is based on an understanding of evidence from applied health care research will provide superior patient care compared with practitioners who rely on understanding of basic mechanisms and their own clinical experience.[32] Regarding the above, I think that an awful lot of assumptions were made.

It was stated that EBM emerged as a reaction toward increasing dissatisfaction with the practice of medicine.

However, a more reliable reason stressing the need for change was that because of the rapid growth of medical knowledge and the widening application of technology, there was a particular need for a continuing authoritative review of both preventive and therapeutic strategies.

At the same time, EBM is not a science of its own but a new branch of medicine, the offspring of statistics, epidemiology and pharmacology which has been generated to help manage a growth of knowledge that is increasingly difficult to cope with.[33]

6. EBM, a nicely framed concept

The term EBM implicitly claims that former clinical medicine, which was not based on meta-analyses or RCTs, was not based on evidence.[31] This seems a kind of implication that the practice of medicine was previously based on direct communication with God or tossing a coin.[26]

But, rightly or wrongly, medicine has always considered itself to be EB. Thus, contemporary advocates of the label 'evidence-based' have chosen an imprecise label – or an arrogant one if they believe their predecessors have not considered their decisions to be EB.[34] Ultimately, any kind of evidence may be combined with clinical expertise, setting, circumstances, patient state, preferences, values and choices.[10] This was always done to a varying degree for all components of practice and decision-making.[10] Medicine has always been evidence-based, only 'evidence' now has taken on a new meaning. The true change is a revision of medical epistemology.[31]

The success of EBM in terms of its dissemination and its proliferation as a slogan or catchphrase can neither be underestimated nor gainsaid.[35] However, such widespread use of a term is not sufficient substantiation of its veracity.[35] Although the term involves a calculatedly dishonest misrepresentation, this new nomenclature was an immediate rhetorical success.[5] EBM effectively labelled itself as rational, objective and altruistic – while any opposition was implied to be promoting a practice that is illogical, self-indulgent and opposed to the evidence.[5] A set of mission-statements was proposed as definitive of EBM: these took the form of platitudes which could not be opposed by any rational person; yet these content-free proclamations served to camouflage controversial ways of operating and marginalize opponents as wicked or crazy.[5] If EBM was a misnomer for 'a service center for literature searches', I would have had nothing against subscribers to the title except perhaps, for a demand to rename themselves to reflect what they actually do or preach to do.[13] But is seems that it was not a poor linguistic choice but rather a carefully selected term.[13]

'Evidence' has a justificatory role. The noun evidence delivers forceful premises of truth.[13] Attempts to upgrade the truth value of some interpretations with the adjective 'systematic' or by classifying some journals as 'evidence-based practice journals' should be regarded as attempts to claim authority over scientific truth.[13] It is offered as a means of supporting conclusions or recommendations to act. Labeling any message as EB is trying to make it automatically more credible in the information consumer's mind.[10] It also erroneously gives proponents that identify with the domain a not sufficiently substantiated feeling of righteousness and power.[10] Even when it is not obligatory to do so, claiming to be 'evidence-based' conveys a measure of credibility nowadays that is valuable to have.[36] Why has it taken defenders of EBM so long to publicly recognize that RCTs are open to manipulation, and that the sobriquet 'EB' is just an attractive prefix to multiple interests?[6]

It is unlikely that the catchphrase of EBM will abate in attractiveness or popularity, as contrary options are not tenable. What could be questionable about the call to practice medicine according to scientific proof or near-proof?[13] Can anyone advocate non-EBM and be considered serious?[13] Who after all would admit to the practice of whimsy-based or inclination-based medicine?[35]

It is perhaps precisely due to its loose meaning that a good number of adherents and followers have become comfortable, enthusiastic and often empowered in this domain.[10] Such vagueness may be a mixed blessing since it has led to disparate domains of problem solving like qualitative research, health economics or management being included within EBM.[10]

Most professional societies, the public and funding agencies have accepted EBM with remarkable enthusiasm. Health care opinion leaders concluded that EBM represents one of the most important medical milestones of the last 160 years, in the same category as innovations such as antibiotics, anesthesia and vaccines.[31,37] Alas, in reality very few real big steps of progression – that would not have occurred without EBM – enriched medical practice the last decades.

So, the term evidence-based is perhaps ill-chosen and occasionally misapplied, and the concept of EBM does take varied forms. Why then do people believe EBM is so straightforward? In the first place, it would be very nice if it were true, and wishful thinking is a powerful impulse.[26] Secondly, there is a profound misunderstanding to the effect that statistics is equated with science.[26] Certainly, the almost magic words 'evidence-based' continue to possess highly persuasive rhetorical force, but it is surely depressing that some colleagues seemingly lack the critical faculties necessary to recognize nonsense in order to expose it for what it is.[24]

"Why is eliminating the use of p-values as a truth so hard? The basic explanation is neither philosophical nor scientific, but sociologic; everyone uses them. It's the same reason we can use money. When everyone believes in something's value, we can use it for real things; Money for food, and p-values for knowledge claims, publication, funding, and promotion. It doesn't matter if the p-value doesn't mean what people think it means; it becomes valuable because of what it buys."[38] I think that substituting EBM for p-values gives the third reason.

It is doubtful whether such a crude, question-begging tactic as naming oneself EBM would have had much influence upon clinicians and medical scientists.[5] However, the proponents of EBM cleverly bypassed doctors and appealed directly to politicians, health service managers, public health professionals and the newly expanded ranks of 'number-crunchers' (epidemiologists, biostatisticians, information technologists, health economists, etc.).[5] EBM was seized upon by managers and their myrmidons, and promoted with a massive injection of publicity, money and organizational infrastructure.[5] The consequence has been an astonishing transformation from the clinically-led approach of CE to the managerially-led approach of EBM.[5]

7. EBM not a new paradigm

A paradigm was defined by Kuhn as a set of scientific and metaphysical beliefs that make up a theoretical framework within which scientific theories can be tested, evaluated, and if necessary revised. When theories, exemplars and standards of the dominant paradigm of the day cannot successfully answer emerging problems in the field, scientific revolution leads to the adoption of a new paradigm.

Probably the biggest mistake (or deliberate action) was made already at the start. The *JAMA* article stated that the change in medical practice which involves using the literature more effectively in guiding medical practice, is profound enough that it can appropriately be called a paradigm shift. So, from its inception, EBM has been envisioned as a 'new paradigm' for the teaching of medicine, a new set of skills and methods of reasoning that allows physicians to incorporate a growing body of medical evidence into practice.[39] However, more effective evaluating literature is not a new way of looking at the world as mentioned by Kuhn. Optimalisation of research assessment and consequently incorporating it more effectively into practice should have been additional to what we had instead of trying to replace it completely.

Promoting better understanding of the principles of epidemiology is not a paradigm shift that necessitates throwing away all other knowledge. Although described as a 'paradigm shift', it really was more of a next stage in the evolution of a focus on critical appraisal of available evidence that had been in progress for years.[36] Only the nature of evidence has changed; a better term fitting the content could have been: 'research enhanced health care'.

According to the EBMWG, EBM requires skills that are not traditionally part of medical training including precisely defining a patient problem.[19] This seems a false accusation; long before I learned about EBM, my first step in practice with the patient was defining the problem. Wasn't precisely defining the problem and what information is required to resolve it, already what doctors were supposed to do? Isn't that why we perform an anamnesis, clinical investigation, and discuss outcomes and expectations? The rest of the skills are especially helpful in case you do not know a solution to the problem. All the times you do know the answer, or on the occasions you did get expert advise the rest of these skills is elaborate and redundant. Most of us do not have time for two critical appraisal exercises per patient.

Clinicians can easily conclude that EBM is not particularly novel, and may wonder why it has stirred so much fuss and controversy.[3] Was clinical epidemiology a new, independent and revolutionary paradigm, seemingly unrelated to its roots? It was not and this should not be the case for EBM either.[11] EBM does not represent a new paradigm, but rather a new name for a still nebulous process called 'clinical medicine'.[39] Or, as Shahar argued: EBM is at best a meaningless substitute for 'medicine' and, at worst, a disguise for a new version of authoritarianism in medical practice.[13]

Describing EBM as a new paradigm, somewhat suggested that the old paradigm, *i.e.*, medical practice as it was, needed to be replaced. But, although improvement of the system might have been necessary, a call for a total replacement is ludicrous. This open challenge to the traditional manner of delivering clinical care and self-characterization of EBM as entirely new and original exemplifies the élan and, some might argue, arrogance of the early pronunciations by its architects.[35]

EBM should not be construed as a new scientific or philosophical theory that changes the nature of medicine or our understanding thereof.[37] Rather, we should consider EBM as a continuously evolving heuristic structure for optimizing clinical practice.[37] Evaluating RCTs and making meta-analysis in a proper way, is just a small additive to the rest of the knowledge. Stressing the importance of proper assessment of evidence from clinical research would have sufficed to ameliorate the overall care. Being critical about 'the way we do things' can be of great help in creating research questions if serious doubt exists. Warning that 'in the absence of systematic observation one must be cautious in the interpretation of information derived from clinical experience and intuition, for it may at times be misleading', might easily cause too much concern. (As demonstrated by Kahneman; human beings are poorly able to make a correct decision under the pressure of uncertainty and fear – *in casu* for being misled – is a bad counselor.)

To the extent that protagonists of the term EBM advocate more reliance on clinical research than on intuition alone, I am fully supportive.[13] Nonetheless, there is nothing new in this paradigm and I see no reason for a new title.[13] Medicine has always been taught and practiced in the light of available scientific experience and interpretation of that scientific experience.[13] Scientific evidence should be integrated in and contrasted with the totality of our beliefs and knowledge. Reasonable doctors never cease to update their medical knowledge.[13]

On the basis of these considerations EBM does not represent a new or special theory of knowledge. In fact, it draws on the major traditions; inference to the best explanation.[37]

8. Criticisms of EBM

EBM is controversial, not because people disagree about whether medical decisions ought to incorporate the best available evidence, but because they disagree about how narrowly evidence is defined.[40]

Unfortunately, EBM has moved directly from being a 'bright idea', to the implementation of this idea – leaving out the usual period of critique, evaluation and testing.[5] EBM enthusiasts see its benefits as self-evident; hence any disagreement is merely indicative of a failure to understand – or else due to a more sinister determination to practice medicine in a non-EB manner.[5] Dissenting views are muzzled, marginalized, met by non-sequiturs, or disappear into an echoing void.[5] But, do we need the burden of numerical proof to support such a self-evidently correct assumption? The answer is, of course, 'Yes'.[41]

EBM involves the elevation of certain methodological principles – in particular the large randomized trial and (more recently) meta-analysis to 'gold standard' status as criteria against which all other types of 'evidence' should be judged.[5] Or, as Norman stated, an essential element of the EBM paradigm is the explicit preoccupation with methodological rigor as a criterion of acceptance or rejection of a particular study.[41] This doctrine excludes or relegates to inferior status the role of implicit or unquantifiable factors such as clinical judgment, experience, qualitative factors, views of patients and the demands of the clinical consultation.[5] Is it in fact the case that the major influences on the bias of the study findings is methodologic quality?[41] Methodological rigor is an insufficient measure of freedom from bias, and other factors – like drug company funding – may lead to greater bias than simply poor study design.[41]

In particular, EBM displays a long-standing tendency towards anti-scientific rhetoric which ignores the foundational role of laboratory and clinical sciences in the history of therapeutic innovation and advance. The misplaced emphasis on large databases as offering best guidance for clinical practice leads on to an implicit belief in the primary role of information and statistics.[5] However, informed decision-making is not simply a matter of straight extrapolation from evidence to decision-making.[41] Consequently, the nature of clinical expertise has been redefined by EBM. It has traditionally been assumed that the best people for deciding upon clinical matters are those with clinical training, experience and a substantive knowledge of health and disease that ideally includes having performed research in the field. Such experts are usually doctors.[5] But EBM regards clinical expertise as mainly a matter of collecting, analyzing and summarizing research done by other people. Hence the final arbiters of EBM practice include 'systematic reviewers' drawn from biostatistics, epidemiology, health economics and other 'infostat' disciplines.[5] Clinical advice has been neatly bypassed and subjected to external performance criteria. This can be regarded as the latest move in an 'audit revolution' which has swept the healthcare sector during the past couple of decades. Suffice it to say that there is not a shred of evidence to suggest that an understanding of medical research and its interpretation for practice can be reduced to the routine application of checklists and formulae.[5] Furthermore, there is no evidence that knowledge gains demonstrated in undergraduate courses in critical appraisal/EBM could be sustained into residency and practice, and eventually could be translated into improved patient outcomes.[41] Moreover, the notion that use of computerized search strategies will readily and efficiently permit access to important clinical research articles is inconsistent with the available data; at least the degree of overlap among expert searchers is much lower than might be supposed.[41]

In a nutshell, EBM involves a takeover of the clinical consultation by an alliance of managers and their statistical technocrats who are empowered to define 'best practice'. The upshot is that the EBM apparatchiks acquire substantive influence over millions of clinical consultations, but without any responsibility for the clinical consequences.[5]

9. EBM and medical practice, what they are and are not.

"EBM is the conscientious, explicit, and judicious use of current best evidence in making decisions about the care of individual patients. The practice of evidence-based medicine means integrating individual clinical expertise with the best available external clinical evidence from systematic research. By individual clinical expertise we mean the proficiency and judgment that individual clinicians acquire through clinical experience and clinical practice. Increased expertise is reflected in many ways, but especially in more effective and efficient diagnosis and in the more thoughtful identification and compassionate use of individual patients' predicaments, rights, and preferences in making clinical decisions about their care."[42] Hardly anyone can disagree with the goal of getting clinicians to make 'conscientious, explicit, and judicious use of current best evidence for decisions in patient care'.[3] The unanswered question is: what is 'best' in each particular circumstance? The best evidence is not available everywhere and there is never enough of it, and we must take this fact into account.[11] Should it not be inference based upon all current evidence instead?

What is conscientious and judicious?

"Good doctors use both individual clinical expertise and the best available external evidence, and neither alone is enough. Without clinical expertise, *practice risks becoming tyrannized by evidence*, for even excellent external evidence may be inapplicable to or inappropriate for an individual patient."[42]

EBM is centered on the notion of the general priority of knowledge obtained by clinical research over other forms of medical knowledge.[39] EBM represents the development, acquisition, critical appraisal and incorporation of a rapidly developing body of evidence into clinical practice.[39] A more restrictive definition: EBM is the process of systematically finding, appraising, and using contemporaneous research findings as the basis for clinical decisions.[10] Or: the consistent use of current best evidence derived from published clinical and epidemiological research in management of patients, with attention to the balance of risks and benefits of diagnostic tests and alternative treatment regimens, taking account of each patient's unique circumstances, including baseline risk, comorbid conditions and personal preferences.[10] A lot of different definitions exist. Most EBM definitions are motivational and persuasive.[10,43] Everyone uses the definition that fits him best. This persistent confusion makes the label EBM divisive.[40]

EBM's understanding of evidence is often perceived as positivist, *i.e.*, recognizing only scientifically verifiable propositions.[10] However, sometimes evidence may be unpublished or indirect, diseases rare, contextual information or resources limited.[7] In these situations, obtaining evidence from experts can be efficient, and experts may be the only or main source of evidence.[7] Expertise is difficult to define and experts do not always agree with one another. Professionals use objective knowledge but also depend on subjective or personal knowledge. Experience frames and elaborates a physician's new case and the cases he shares with other physicians. Over time, experience builds the doctor's capacity to subject experiential data to personal reasoning. To say that knowledge is subjective is not to say that it is arbitrary, un-rigorous, or ineffective.[16] Subjective knowledge is arguably more powerful than statistical analysis, and more experienced professionals possess greater subjective knowledge.[16] Pattern recognition entails immersion in particular situations, past and present, and myriad, sometimes unconscious, determinations about important similarities and differences between particulars.[16]

Medical practice requires that we interpret data from studies, not that we apply a fixed answer.[27] Reliance on expert opinion is not an unfortunate consequence of an underdeveloped EBM but a necessary requirement for the optimal practice of clinical medicine.[44]

For professionals, their work is an act of interpretation that moves back and forth between the general and the particular and among particulars.[16] Interpretation does not assume, as application does, that the individual is most clearly seen as a member of a group.[16] The value of expert opinion lies both in its ability to define the context in which clinical science is undertaken and the help it provides in overcoming the epistemic gap that exists between the results of clinical research and the care of individual patients. Many self-declared practitioners of EBM often do not warn the intended audience about applying the results of a well-designed study of an intervention evaluated in a narrowly defined group of patients to a much broader group of patients who differ from the study group in clinically meaningful ways. Evidence itself is not sufficient, but requires a set of extra or non-evidential considerations. These can only be made by doctors practicing medicine. In other words, much of the work of making decisions and implementing policies requires the necessary integration of these diverse considerations.

EBM requires new skills of the physician, including efficient literature searching and the application of formal rules of evidence evaluating the clinical literature. Still, intuition is very useful at some points in patient care, and it can be of great importance to know pathophysiology, anatomy, farmacotherapy, and so on, as well as having a lot of unsystematic clinical experience. Most of us would prefer the expertise that comes from experience guided by evidence, rather than by guidelines and evidence alone.[27] If I have a car accident, I rather have a well-trained experienced surgeon using some of his intuition as caregiver than a resident with a library.

Expert opinion does not belong in the rankings of the quality of empirical evidence because it does not represent a form of empirical evidence.[44] Expert opinion demands a separate place in a more inclusive medical epistemology than that described by EBM thus far.[44]

The clinician's appeal to a local expert for assistance represents an attempt to broaden the base of experiential knowledge available to aid decision making. The expert's experiential knowledge is not fundamentally different in kind compared with that possessed by the individual clinician, but would be expected to be a richer and more complete version, given the expert's exposure to a larger number of patients of a certain type.[44] Becoming an expert involves learning to use scientific knowledge and medical evidence in clinical-decision making. Expertise means that clinicians can actually justify, and thus be held accountable for their decisions. Doctors have a professional responsibility to come up with the best possible diagnosis and treatment plan for individual patients.[45]

To meet this responsibility, the key epistemological challenge of doctors involves gathering and integrating all relevant, yet heterogeneous sources of information, including not just scientific-medical knowledge of diseases and treatments and diagnostic data on the patient, but also contextual information so as to construct a coherent 'picture' of the patient's disease and its possible treatments.[45]

Instead of deferring responsibility to general clinical guidelines, as at least some interpretations of EBM suggest, doctors should consider themselves epistemologically responsible for producing good quality diagnosis and treatment.[45]

10. Applying evidence

Evidence is not synonymous with truth, but rather serves as a type of justification for certain claims.

Critical appraisal as we know it, that is, of evidence itself, is not critical appraisal of the thinking process in which already critically appraised evidence is applied.[11]

How strong the evidence should be when making a particular type of decision should depend on the consequences of drawing a wrong conclusion.[36] To start with in medicine, a wrong conclusion can be disastrous for the patient. Other important factors are the cost of intervening, the magnitude of potential improvement in health outcome relative to the cost of the intervention (cost-effectiveness), and who is paying for the intervention.[36] A variety of types of evidence might be weighed to come to the conclusion that the risks associated with a product are 'acceptable' compared with the demonstrated benefits of the product. For example, many chemotherapies are very toxic, but their side effects are deemed acceptable when considered in light of their benefits.[36]

The laudable goal of making clinical decisions based on evidence can be impaired by the restricted quality and scope of what is collected as 'best available evidence'.[3] A more inclusive model of evidence has been proposed that stresses the importance of context in the creation of evidence and places equal weight on qualitative and quantitative sources of evidence.[9] EBM would supposedly make medical knowledge central to ethical medical practice in a rather strong way and also uses stringent criterion for what should count as medical knowledge. Proponents are throwing sand in the eyes of their critics by adopting a persistently anti-authoritarian stance which serves to conceal the fact that they are setting themselves up as new authority figures who have taken upon themselves the right to define evidence and its interpretation. Protagonists of EBM who continue to herald EBM as the new medical orthodoxy, seemingly believing that real, good and competent medicine has only recently been discovered, still exist.[46] Instead of being seen as only one of many tools to alleviate suffering and focus on the meaning of illness, researchers adopting a positivist perspective believe that it is the sole means of achieving progress and more cost-effective healthcare.[25]

The sharp distinction between objective and subjective ways of reasoning enshrined in the epistemology of EBM are inappropriate for understanding the epistemology of actual clinical practice.[45] In medical practice, doctors are held accountable both for the gathering of relevant information and for how they fit this information together. This does not only involve the rule-based reasoning of EBM.[45]

Evidence can be used in varying circumstances, for example: (a) the evidence of effectiveness challenge; (b) the authority challenge; (c) the conflicting hierarchy challenge; (d) the definition of evidence challenge.[35]

Ad a: What is the evidence that EBM provides superior clinical care and that its practitioners have better clinical outcomes?

Ad b: What secures the authority of appraisers and disseminators of evidence? There are no standards of accreditation or quality control for those who appraise evidence and disseminate it. In essence we have the replacement of one system of authority with another.

Ad c: Practitioners from backgrounds in the social sciences and humanities (to say nothing of law) may differ with colleagues in clinical epidemiology in their conceptualization of evidence.[35] It is for this reason that alternative models of evidence have been proposed that attempt to accommodate both meaning and measurement, the particular and the general aspect of context, in order to create different modes of evidence that would incorporate both the qualitative and quantitative dimensions of decision making.[35] It is crucial to understand certain properties of evidence and what purpose evidence serves in clinical decision making.[35]

Ad d: EBM's definition of evidence is reductive and far too restrictive and fails to admit a broad range of inputs that should be part of the deliberation of reason. It is hardly surprising that the term is confusing to many who do not appreciate that its evidence is narrowly defined as having to do with systematic observations from certain types of research.[35]

11. Ever changing meaning and explanation of the concept

Correct definitions of any subject of interest are crucial for our understanding and for a subsequent validity of the argumentation we use to solve problems and to determine what is part of the subject and what is not.[10] In case of EBM, we may not be entirely sure what it is that is being proposed, but the language in which the proposal is couched reassures us, that whatever it is, it must be very reasonable.[43]

Ambiguous and vague definitions hamper clear thinking. The greater the number of definitions of a particular subject, the greater our persisting uncertainty regarding the subject.[10] Do we have a clear answer as to what EBM is today?[10] The thing I find odd is that its keenest defenders do not seem to be very clear on this.[43]

After all these years of development and practice, EBM itself needs to be redefined to reflect its present orientation, dimension and scope.[10]

Like the OM, EBM began by stating a clear and explicit preference for empirical evidence, defined as evidence derived from formal and systematic clinical research, over alternate kinds of medical knowledge, specifically individual clinical expertise, expert opinion and pathophysiologic rationale as grounds for medical decision-making.[21]

The EBMWG stated it did not bear nihilism in mind: the criteria should not be presented in a way that fosters nihilism (if the study is not randomized, it is useless and provides no valuable information), but as a way of helping arrive at the strength of inference associated with a clinical decision.[19] Serial refinements to the original definition were forthcoming.[35] EBM began to call for the integration of some alternate kinds of medical knowledge as well as patient goals and values into clinical decision-making.[21] More recently, the focus has shifted to integrating clinical expertise, pathophysiologic knowledge and patient preferences in making decisions regarding the care of individual patients.[39] These shifts mark a critical and necessary recognition of the value of alternative forms of medical knowledge and reasoning.[39] Defined so broadly, there is certainly not a physician alive who would not claim to practice EBM; we physicians strive to use all our knowledge, in its various forms, to benefit our patients.[39]

The EBMWG was well aware of the fact that clinical experience and the development of clinical instincts (particularly with respect to diagnosis) are a crucial and necessary part of becoming a competent physician.[19] Many aspects of clinical practice cannot, or will not, ever be adequately tested.[19] Clinical experience and its lessons are particularly important in these situations.[19] Furthermore, the EBMWG wanted to decrease emphasis, but ascertained that it "didn't imply a rejection of what one can learn from colleagues and teachers, whose years of experience have provided them with insight into methods of history taking, physical examination, and diagnostic strategies. This knowledge can never be gained from formal scientific investigation. EBM also involves applying traditional skills of medical training. A sound understanding of pathophysiology is necessary to interpret and apply the results of clinical research".[19] The shift from 'de-emphasizing' towards 'integrating' alternative forms of medical knowledge and reasoning represents a recognition of the intrinsic gap between research and practice.[39,44]

Proponents of EBM have acknowledged the importance of experiential knowledge in the form of the individual clinician's experience, but currently refuse to give credence to the value of expert opinion.[44] This resistance appears to be necessary to support the claim that EBM represents a novel approach to clinical medicine.[44]

According to Karanicolas *et al.*: "… wise use of the literature requires a sophisticated hierarchy of evidence. Finally, evidence alone is never sufficient to make clinical decisions; rather it requires trading of benefits and risks, inconvenience, and costs, and in doing so considering patients' values and preferences."[47]

The introduction of sophistication entails a contrast or differentiation between the true EBM hierarchy and less sophisticated or cruder hierarchies.[6] Introducing the notion of wise use of literature, though entirely appropriate and justified, does not secure the soundness of EBM's scientific base, but actually moves it away from a vision of science rooted in statistical and epidemiological approaches.[6] Although I agree wholeheartedly with recognizing the importance of wisdom in medical decision-making, I fail to see how wisdom is part of the scientific basis of EBM.[6]

A method for integrating evidence with patient's values and preferences has not been clearly stated except that clinical judgement and expertise are viewed as essential for success.[40] Similarly, concern for judgements, trade-offs between risk and benefits, and incremental costs are not the sort of things (for the most part) whose justification can come from SRs or RCTs.[6] When looking for a deeper account for the justification of EBM, one is drawn away from predominantly scientific accounts and towards justifications that draw on ethical considerations.[6] The status of such concepts needs to be argued for and embedded in a justification, rather than bluntly asserted. Explicitness and transparency function prominently in the justification and these are important and laudable qualities.[6] Yet they are not self-evident, nor easily derived from principles of EBM.[6] These developments indicate a new vison of EBM, one radically different from its origins.

The initial EBM doctrines, so set in stone as absolutes at the time, are now in ruins, such that it is currently difficult to define quite what those colleagues who still describe themselves as 'evidence-based practitioners' actually now believe in.[24]

The latest developments within EBM appear to acknowledge that the universal set of rules that govern medical evidence may not be possible to develop.[37] Instead, the focus has shifted to transparency and explicitness in interpretation of evidence and making recommendations.[37] In essence, the means by which EBM now seeks ultimate justification is by appealing to its trustworthiness.

12. EBM has never been tested in the way it should have been

Where is the evidence about the superiority of EBM practice?[10]

That EBM produces better outcomes is one of its regulating assumptions. Many remarks in the literature describing the foundation of EBM, like the famous work by Archibald Cochrane himself, and by the EBMWG are based on assumptions: "the suggestions made here may not be perfect but I believe they are on the right lines"; "House staff believe that"; "we believe that…"; "a final assumption of the new paradigm is that physicians whose practice is based on an understanding of the underlying evidence will provide superior patient care".[19,28]

For a movement such as EBM to claim legitimacy or even superiority, however, there must be positive arguments to provide its justification, and these must advance beyond proclamation of correctness, popularity, or endorsement by others.[35] No one has run a controlled trial comparing EBM performance with some other best possible intervention or model of care yet. Thus, EBM has failed so far to provide the evidence that it does more good, than harm. EBM is unsuccessful in providing scientific evidence for its own utility in improving the process and outcome of clinical care. EBM is indeed, a belief, conviction or claim that still must be fully justified.[10] It is not clear whether it will ultimately benefit patients. Even the EBMWG recognized this problem: "Our advocating evidence-based medicine in the absence of definitive evidence of its superiority in improving patient outcomes may appear to be an internal contradiction."[19] Ironically, if one were to develop guidelines for how to teach EBM based on these results, they would be based on the lowest level of evidence.[48] The most frequently reported outcomes are subjective variables such as satisfaction or self-reported changes in attitude or knowledge, rather than more important assessments of objective measured clinical skills or improved patient outcomes.[48]

Evaluation whether physicians practice EBM well and consistently still does not mean automatically that their performance yields better results.[10] We need evidence of EBM's effectiveness. Otherwise, following EBM's philosophy remains just another new belief, regardless of how intellectually justified it might be. Our sincere belief (confidence in the truth or existence of EBM's superiority not immediately susceptible to rigorous proof) or conviction as a fixed or firm belief in the soundness of EBM is still not enough to advance EBM farther.[10] According to EBMWG: the proof of the pudding is no more achievable for the new paradigm than it is for the old, for no long-term randomized trials of traditional medicine and EBM are likely to be carried out.[19] This is a curious concession, particularly for a method that upholds empirical evidence as the most compelling justification for belief and action.[35]

So, although it all seems logical, there is little evidence about this alleged improvement of medical care especially if 'evidence' is used in the nihilistic way. It is inconceivable that we keep on going on this path, as long as the question of whether the practice of EBM produces better results than its alternatives, remains unanswered and despite the lack of good evidence that teaching EBM improves the quality of medical education or the subsequent care of patients. The justification of EBM by stressing its spread, wide acceptance and practice by many is an *ad populum* fallacy.[10]

The initial creation of an evidence hierarchy was intended to link the quality of evidence to the soundness of the recommendations based on the evidence. However, once again a great irony exists because the entire edifice of evidence hierarchies is not based on systematic research at all, but on expert judgement or consensus. In other words, the warrant or justification for viewing evidence in such a hierarchical structure, rests on the lowest form of evidence, that is the beliefs of a few.[35]

Thus, EBM is currently to be seen as a 'form' or 'mode' of clinical practice, theoretical and experimental in nature, with no evidence whatsoever for a superior clinical effectiveness or patient satisfaction profile.[24]

With these quite central and fundamental objections documented, and supported by an extensive literature, it seems extraordinary that so much argument continues to take place, that so many medical education curricula continue to change with reference to EBM criteria, and that so much clinical practice has been altered – all on the basis of a concept underpinned by an absolute lack of evidentiary basis.[24]

While it may not be easy to devise a rigorous study of EBM, it is incumbent on the practitioners of EBM to provide leadership and do their best, if their appeals that clinical practice should be based primarily on 'best research evidence' to ring true.[41] According to the proponents, no such evidence is available from randomized trials because no investigative team has yet overcome the problems of sample size, contamination and blinding that such a trial raises. In my opinion this constitutes a *testimonium paupertatis*; given the importance of the subject they should have tried a lot harder!

And actually, if anyone wants to run this trial, I can come up with a couple of topics, that I am quite sure of, will lead to better outcomes both objectively and subjectively if treated with a combination of the best available evidence from literature and guidelines with my expertise than if treated only with best available evidence from literature and guidelines.

The EBMWG stated that withholding access to evidence from the control arm in such a trial would be unethical. However, the control arm should exist of doctors applying 'all evidence' instead of the so called supposedly 'best research evidence' only; so there would be no such thing as 'withholding'.

On the contrary, I would like to argue that withholding therapies only because no RCTs exist is unethical!

13. What does a doctor-patient relation look like?

Understanding the goals, values, and preferences of the individual patient are necessary to any determination about what kind of medical intervention should be offered.[38] EBM failed to appreciate and cultivate this complex nature of sound clinical judgement. On the contrary, because of its reliance on population-derived evidence, EBM drives (indeed, requires) the clinician to reason from the general to the particular, which cuts across traditional clinical assessment and management which runs from the particular to the general.[49] Unfortunately, the effort, expense and apparent rigor of the guideline development process place the clinician under substantial pressure to adhere to them.[49]

Rarely, however, do physicians defend clinical autonomy on philosophical grounds by arguing that multifaceted medical knowledge is a better basis for patient care than even the most rigorous aggregate outcome data.[18] Professional judgement is not in itself a type of evidence but rather it is a means for adjudicating between alternative sources and weighing their relevance to the problem at hand.[1] Physicians should assert the legitimacy – indeed the necessity – of reasoning about individual patients on the basis of personal experience and theories of cause and effect, as well as on the basis of statistical knowledge.[18] The knowledge that a procedure is more or less effective overall should not be confused with the knowledge of whether or how to use that procedure in caring effectively for the next patient.[18] Even the best clinical science is less than all of what physicians know.[18]

Medical knowledge involves many ways of knowing. Medical knowledge is more like deliberation than like calculation, insightful as well as informed, a gestalt or story rather than an algorithm.[18]

The clinical science of OR, as informative as it is, cannot substitute for either clinical expertise or clinical sense.[18] It is not enough to know the average benefit of treatment.[27] We need to know for which patient, under what conditions, treated for how long, and with what other therapies a given strategy is best.[27] Care of patients is an act, not of application of guidelines, but of interpretation of information.[18,27] The art of medicine includes interpreting data, not simply applying them. Not all questions of relevance to the care of patients are scientific in their nature and so science cannot ever provide the basis for clinical decision-making in any fundamental sense.

Medicine needs a more robust epistemology capable of recognizing patients and clinicians as persons.[40] A person-centered medical epistemology requires a revised conception of medical uncertainty and a recognition that clinician-patient interactions are central to medicine.[40]

Tacit knowing refers to the taken-for-granted knowledge at the periphery of attention that allows people to understand the world and discern meaning in it.[40] A good doctor pays explicit attention to the patient's story, while simultaneously being aware of the patient's tone of voice, facial expressions, and choice of words.[40] Explicit awareness of one observation always depends on and presupposes tacit awareness of many others, but attempts to bring tacit or background observations into explicit focus disrupts understanding of the original event.[40]

All human knowledge has a practical dimension rooted in the accretions of experience and memory.[40] Infants learn to speak without structured training, children learn to ride bicycles with only cursory instruction and medical students learn to identify diseases without memorizing diagnostic algorithms.[40] Tacit knowing is not some mystical ability; it is a consequence of how humans interact with reality.[40] Human beings accrue knowledge tacitly through experience and observation and make decisions that take tacit knowing into account.[40]

When a clinician shifts his or her focus from a patient's story to a patient's words, the words come into explicit focus, but the meaning of the story necessarily recedes into the background.[40] Tacit knowing is certainly not infallible, and misleading tacit knowing is, by its nature, harder to recognize than faulty conclusions from clinical trials or clinical experience[40] (and causes doctors to do the same stupid thing over and over again).

Therefore, improving feedback to clinical practitioners may be the most effective debiasing procedure available.

However, EBM proponents mistakenly identify tacit knowing with the 'opinion and unsystematic clinical experience' their movement was designed to supplant.[40]

Clinicians do not make decisions by reckoning objective data and clinical probabilities; rather they reach decisions in light of the particular tacit and explicit data they recover while encountering their patients as persons.[40] Clinicians usually fail to note the tacit component of medical reasoning because they appropriately focus on helping patients rather than on analyzing their own thought processes, just as they focus on patients' stories rather than on patients' exact spoken words.[40]

Clinical decisions are made through a plurality of means and are formulated on the basis of what quite non-seductively be termed evidence of the clinic, constituted not only by the randomized controlled trial but from a variety of other sources, including raw clinical experience, complex patient biography, a telling phrase, even an inadvertent gesture.[46,50]

The more pragmatic vision of the clinical encounter expressed by informal logic may resonate with clinicians' experience as it places patient values, clinical experience, and clinical research on equal grounds.[9]

Trust in clinical relationship may have a subsidiary effect of reinforcing the unearned authority of doctors, but trust is far more than this.[26] Indeed, trust is intrinsic to a proper clinical relationship – it is not some kind of 'bolt-on' optional extra, insisted upon by doctors against the patient's wishes. Doctors do not claim the right to be trusted; rather patients want a doctor whom they can trust.[26] Without trust the consultation cannot function properly.

Although patients want 'effective' treatment, and doctors should strive to discover effective treatments and ensure that patients receive them, effectiveness is not the sole item of medical practice. Patients will continue to demand the consultation as 'the essential unit' of medical practice – they will seek explanation, prognostication, reassurance, advice…

in other words they will seek a personal clinical relationship.[26]

The proper goal for clinical practice is to build upon a basis of genuinely rigorous science, honed with epidemiological measurement where its use is valid and applicable.[26] The core of clinical medicine is, and should remain, the provision of personal medical services by means of consultation. And the place of EBM must be subordinate to this.[26]

14. Public Health versus individual care

The OM and consequently EBM caused a shift in focus from the individual to society at large.

However, the optimal health of each individual is not identical with the optimal health of the group, and the duty of the clinician may conflict with the duty of the public health doctor.[51] Interventions offering the possibility of great benefits to the nation may offer only a minuscule chance to benefit to, or actually harm, individual people.[51] For health plans, achieving the best outcomes for the population of patients is the principal objective, whereas physicians' principal obligation is to achieve the best clinical outcome for individual patients.

A health care intervention is considered to be 'efficacious' when there is evidence that the intervention is beneficial when administered by experts in a research setting.[36] An intervention is considered 'effective' when there is evidence that it is beneficial when administered by a representative sample of physicians in routine practice settings to the full spectrum of patients to whom provided; so, if it is beneficial in real life.[36]

Clinical medicine is fundamentally a prudential and personal discipline, relating one individual in need of healing with another, who professes and promises to heal.[39] It represents an attempt to improve or maintain the health of an individual.[39] Public health aims to benefit society at large by improving health across populations.[39] Certainly not mutually exclusive, but they are distinct goals that, at times, come into conflict.[39] The direct application of knowledge derived from population-based studies is likely to fulfill the goal of public health; the application of the same knowledge to the individual, is problematic.[39] Moreover, due to all kinds of restrictions, for example insurance companies who do not refund specific types of therapy because of a supposed lack of evidence, individualized patient care might even be worse if based on public health issues.

Governments around the world are rejoicing in the growth of the EBM religion because it makes it easier to withhold or withdraw support from all forms of care for which there is deemed to be insufficient evidence.[52] Unfortunately, most current medical epistemologies do not recognize qualitative differences among clinician-patient medical decisions, healthcare system management decision, health care payor decisions, and population-level public health policy decisions.

In EBM, the individuality of patients tends to be devalued, the focus of clinical practice is subtly shifted away from the care of the individuals toward the care of populations, and the complex nature of sound clinical judgement is not fully appreciated.[38] The attraction of such an approach for politicians and governments committed to reducing the 'burden' of public expenditure is not hard to fathom.[25] Increasingly doctors will be reduced to performing 'cookbook medicine' involving the technical application of clinical guidelines based on largely economic criteria.[25] The OM is ascendant now in many universities, government agencies, research organizations and in the market place. EBM is now siding with insurance agencies, public and private, and their budget-cutting administrators, as procedures unsupported by full 'evidence' might someday soon, be no longer reimbursed.[33] However, EBM – if it is what it claims to be – should ally itself first to the practicing doctor, and only afterwards offer clinically sound advice to third party payers.[33]

EBM feeds a very modern craving for explicitness concerning method. This craving is a consequence of the increased role of management in contemporary society, which carries with it an inner dynamic for imposing bureaucratic systems – and bureaucracy can only control what is explicit.[26] Explicitness is therefore typically regarded as more important than validity.[26]

The distinctive spin that EBM put on this question of variations in practice and outcomes is concerned not so much with causes – about which EBM is agnostic – as with solutions.[26] If variations are a problem, then enforced uniformity is the solution, and EBM claims the ability to determine which uniformity ought to be enforced.[26] The trouble is that for every case of variations that has been uncovered and rolled forward triumphantly for inspection by the protagonists of EBM, the would be clear-cut guidelines as to EBM recommendations are almost invariable found to be partial and controversial at best, and inappropriate and hazardous at worst.[26] Low adherence to even seemingly straightforward guidelines can result from patients' particular circumstances rather than poor care.[40]

It is only by ignoring or down-grading the importance of the many other variables which feed into clinical decisions, and by concentrating exclusively on data such as RCTs, that the illusory clarity of EB standard practice can be achieved. EBM displays a marked propensity to count and measure which can only reinforce a dependence on biomedical positivism with all its attendant flaws and limitations.[25]

EBM stands revealed as statistical rather than scientific; its success has more to do with managerial dominance than medical desirability.[5] Any modest initial benefits have long since been outweighed by structural damage, wasted expenditure, and clinical power without clinical responsibility.[5]

EBM has advanced audit into the consultation, and offers the prospect of an EB health service forcibly unified under a single 'quality assurance' system – easily regulated by politicians, bureaucrats and their statistical technicians.[5] Administrative decisions to limit the quality of care to reduce costs should be admitted fairly instead of pretending that 'best practice' and 'most cost-effective' are synonyms.[40] It is not surprising, then, that mistrust arises in those contexts where perception of the capacity to do harm, usually in the face of some organizational or impersonal body, outweighs any perception of benefit.[6] Clinical guidelines and protocols, developed under the guise of helping doctors practice better medicine, could actually become instruments of control.[25] We shall be left with an outcome which EBM is intended to address, namely, arbitrary, *ad hoc* rationing; but this time based on fashion and the whims of managers and their advisers.

15. A hierarchy of evidence does not exist

In EBM, standardized methods are available for the classification of the evidential level of research. The hierarchy implies that empirical evidence, especially when of high quality should be viewed as so compelling as to obviate the need to consider clinical experience or physiologic understanding in a clinical decision.

The assertion that empirical evidence derived from clinical research, when present, always provides 'better evidence' to guide clinical decision-making is erroneous.[21] Each potential source of medical knowledge carries with it a different complement of strengths and weaknesses. The notion that evidence can be reliably placed in hierarchies is illusory, as stated by Rawlins. According to him, decision-makers need to assess and appraise all the available evidence irrespective of whether it has been derived from randomized controlled trials or observational studies; the strengths and weaknesses of each need to be understood if reasonable and reliable conclusions are to be drawn.[53] It will be up to the properly trained practitioner to assess the merits of different sources of evidence in the specific context of her/his practice, taking into account many considerations – including, in many medical encounters, the goals of patients and the views of colleagues as well as sources of published research.[1]

Or, as even Sackett and Wennberg admitted, each method should flourish, because each has features that overcome the limitations of the others when confronted with questions they cannot reliably answer.[54] As a consequence, there is no invariant hierarchy of evidence that can be applied in each context, and the need to pursue research evidence will therefore vary accordingly.[9]

A hierarchy of evidence is not something observable in the natural world nor in any sense axiomatic.[6] The idea of a hierarchy itself is not derived from the types of reasoning at the top of the hierarchy.[6] Ancillary arguments need to be made independent of the hierarchy to explain why evidence can be regarded hierarchically, and why the particular hierarchy proposed by EBM is in any way superior to other candidates.[6] The arguments for the hierarchy rest on concerns for the mitigation of certain biases, such as selection and observer bias.

The hierarchy of evidence is based essentially on the methodological character of studies rather than on their quality.[10] The current hierarchy is based mainly on the theoretical nature of each study contributing to the demonstration of some cause-effect relationship wherever experimental proof (clinical trial) is possible.[10] It presumes implicitly that any clinical trial is automatically and by definition better than any other kind of cause-effect link demonstration like observational analytical studies.[10] It is as if the mere adherence to any explicit and pre-determined algorithm carries an automatic superiority. But a flawed clinical trial is, of course, not superior to an impeccable observational analytical study.[10] A poorly designed study that is high in the preceding hierarchy may well be more susceptible to bias than a well-designed study that is lower.[36]

All available evidence constitutes far more than just trials or other research results. EBM has struggled with the value and integration of other kinds of medical knowledge such as those derived from clinical experience or based on pathophysiologic rationale. The assignment of these kinds of knowledge to the lower rungs of the hierarchy of evidence are, of course, not evidence-based themselves, but rather represent philosophical (more precisely, epistemological) assertions.[21] However, the general priority given to empirical evidence derived from clinical research in all EBM approaches is not epistemically tenable.[21] Empirical evidence, experiential evidence and pathophysiological understanding differ in kind from one another, not in degree.[21] Therefore, these cannot be placed in the same hierarchy and should be used next to each other. What these various kinds of knowledge do share is the potential to serve as warrants for clinical decisions.[21]

What is more important in research synthesis: is it an overall impression based on all quantitative analysis refinements that methodological perfectionism might provide (sometimes teasingly referred to as PhD syndrome), or is it a rational analysis and interpretation of the meaning and applicability of a mosaic of original studies as an epidemiology of their results, however heterogeneous they might be?[10] Critical appraisal of evidence comprises more in-depth reasoning; which is the best, which is acceptable and which should be discarded? How strong a source of evidence is expert opinion versus a well-conducted cohort study of 500 patients versus a somewhat flawed clinical trial of 200 patients?[55]

Experiential evidence encompasses the knowledge gained from the direct care of patients.[21] The practicing doctor may rely on personal experience or attempt to learn from the personal experience of others.[21] With experiential knowledge, more is generally considered better than less.[21] Hence expert opinion, when based on extensive experience with large numbers of patients with a particular disease, may be viewed as the highest form of experiential evidence.[21] The major problem with experiential knowledge is that it is prone to multiple kinds of cognitive bias, with potentially false conclusions about causality or treatment effect being drawn.[21]

Expertise is acquired by repeated practice and feedback especially about mistakes. It vividly demonstrates the difference between propositional knowledge, acquired in the early years of medical education, and the practical know-how acquired by post-graduate medical education and experience.[56] It emphasizes the role of prior clinical experience.

It is easy enough to organize studies according to a hierarchy of methodological rigor, but where is the logical demarcation between evidence and no evidence?[13] Between weak evidence and strong evidence?[13] When is there 'enough evidence' to practice EBM and when is there not?[13] In some cases, all doctors would make the same decision; in many others they would differ.[11]

A casuistic alternative to EBM recognizes that five distinct topics are potentially relevant to any clinical decision: (1) empirical evidence; (2) experiential evidence; (3) pathophysiologic rationale; (4) patient goals and values; and (5) system features.[21] No general priority exists, relative importance depends upon circumstances.

If non-evidentiary forms of medical knowledge are given equal status to empirical evidence, then the primary axiom of EBM, which identifies research-derived evidence as the 'best evidence' to guide clinical decision making, is undermined.[21] If non-evidentiary knowledge is allowed to trump empirical evidence, then the clinician who knows and understands the clinical research relevant to a particular condition but chooses to treat patients with that condition in a manner not supported by the empirical evidence can still claim to be practicing 'EBM', as he is simply integrating clinical experience in a conscientious, explicit and judicious fashion that happens to give priority to that experience.[21]

16. Research and practice

"In theory, theory and practice are the same, in practice they are not."
– A. Einstein

Clinical experience seems to be quite different from clinical research. The former is direct and personal, the latter indirect and general.[21] In fact, a classic philosophical distinction exists between first-hand, primary experience and empirical evidence derived from systematic observation and experimentation, the so called 'processed information'.[21]

Alas, advocates of EBM may often be diverted from the bedside to the library or computer terminal.[3] Looking up the literature in a systematic fashion is very time-consuming for anybody who looks after patients.[33] After all, the computer boys of EBM spend weeks and weeks doing just that.[33] Clinicians, resentfully, feel watched by nerds who spend their time sipping coffee while talking to computers instead of patients.[33] Increasingly since doctors are not only being advised on how to organize and interpret the results of their research work, which makes sense, but are also told what to do in everyday practice, which is the bone of contention.[33] All the more so, as self-appointed controllers have sprung from totally different walks of life, EBM should resist temptations to regulate the rest of medicine. Applying guidelines is not as straightforward as some may like to think.[33] The main focus in medicine is the patient, not the evidence.

Training in biostatistics and clinical epidemiology has led to the production of medical experts whose expertise is not in any particular aspect of clinical practice, but in study design and interpretation.[44] EBM makes important claims about both the theory and practice of medicine.[37] EBM makes a normative claim about when some kinds of medical knowledge can genuinely be taken as knowledge.[37] However, there is room for dispute regarding the design of a study on the grounds of measurement error, contaminated solution, malfunctioned equipment, poor design, or bias. So, even within the confines of strictly EBM practice, empirical evidence undergoes numerous subjective interpretations. Maier described by way of specific example the limited validity of psychiatric diagnoses and notes how EBM, which is fundamentally based on correctness of diagnosis has an almost automatically doubtful applicability in psychological medicine.[57]

Although a literature search is supposed to be 'systematic', I doubt that a guideline based on a non-systematic review will lead to an outcome very different from a systematic one. It is hard to believe that the outcome would be totally different because one (or a couple of) influential article(s) would not be retrieved and were unknown to the experts who write the review or guideline. Moreover, systematic reviewing might seem highly logical, however, it is conditional on two constraints: (1) all evidence needs to be in the literature; and (2) all levels of evidence must be evaluated. In most cases both constraints are not met. Medical journals are littered by iterating papers on fashionable lines of investigation while genuinely interesting results, be they unexpected or simply negative, fall foul of negative publication bias.[33]

I think that a guideline written by experts in the field and supported by literature will be a far more useful document than many current guidelines that are based on a systematic review of trials only. This because many diagnostic topics as well as treatments/therapies are lost if only trials are reviewed. Consequently, many (especially young) colleagues who adhere to the guidelines and do not have sufficient knowledge to deviate from them, will lack part of the medical armamentarium because of the overly restricted guideline content.

Empiricists build probabilistic models depicting the likelihood of relationships between phenomena but not to the reasons for these relationships.[16] By comparison, realism pursues what actually is and builds determinist models of cause and effect.[16] An approach to EBM which adopts an unswerving faith in scientific positivism reinforces the belief that 'reality' consists only of phenomena that can be quantified and measured.[25]

Increased attention to the principles of EBM among policy makers and purchasers should lead to the preservation of funding for proven efficacious therapies and elimination only of interventions that have been shown to be harmful or ineffective. That statement might be nice in theory, but nowadays, in practice everything 'not proven by trials' is not reimbursed because insurance companies state that no evidence exists. In the Netherlands, in ENT practice, this holds true for example for tuba dilation and hyperbaric oxygen for sudden deafness (just to mention a few of the enormous amount of thrown-away therapies). So, in theory proponents can claim that they were never nihilistic, but EBM is practiced in a nihilistic way by many of the self-proclaimed EBM doctors.

17. Reasoning about evidence

Making justified decisions is more complex and refined than the rule-based reasoning that EBM theory promotes. Doctors have a responsibility to (1) gather and use relevant information and knowledge; (2) employ different types of reasoning for specific situations; and (3) make the intellectual effort to use these types of knowledge and reasoning so as to come up with good diagnoses and treatment plans that fit with current perceptions of best practice.[45] Please note that 'the best' evidence is only meaningful if used in proper argumentation.[10] Clinical experience often, but not always, equals compatibility with evidence. Let us not forget that the by far greatest amount of evidence does not stem from RCTs; how many spoken sentences do you need to hear to judge whether or not a speaker is a native or a non-native speaker?[56]

Reasoning consists of several overlapping phases (a) collecting sensations and observations – what we might call data; (b) interpreting those data and leading hopefully to understanding; (c) weighing up competing interpretations by a process of judgement; and (d) choosing how to act (what is the right thing to do) – a process of deliberation.[17] This reasoning should be reflexive and informed by scientific evidence – but the latter can never replace the former.

Argumentation is a process of proposing, defining and explaining, and valuing considerations designed to support and justify some claim.[11] Doctors may differ in their final assessments based on the weight they give to different potential warrants, but they must be aware of and fully consider the empirical evidence available in reaching conclusions.[21] I concur with the statement that medical reasoning must be rigorous and explicit. What might otherwise appear to be simply differences in style or opinion on the part of clinicians can be made explicit and traced back to differences in the weight given to conflicting warrants.[21] As such, the root causes of practice variability can be made clear.[21]

The personal and prudential nature of clinical decision-making means that clinicians may reasonably differ in assessments, conclusions, and recommendations regarding the care of individual patients.[21] The optimal practice of clinical medicine, although requiring the knowledge of the results of clinical research, demands that doctors thoughtfully consider both evidentiary and non-evidentiary warrants for action in each attempt to deliver the best care to a particular individual.[21]

Understanding basic biological and physiological principles allows doctors to relate presenting features to a diagnosis and to anticipate and measure response to therapy. The strength of pathophysiological reasoning primarily depends on the strength of the underlying biological or physiological theory.[21]

A critical dimension of clinical judgement is knowing (at least at an intuitive level) which patients to manage using fast thinking (based on crude classification) and which require us to revert to slow thinking (individualized management).[49] When does the physician need to engage in a slow, careful logical process of hypotheses generation and testing, and when will short-cut methods, like pattern recognition or recalling the solution to a previous case work just as well or better?[56] Or, are time pressure and economics determining that quick, simple methods will dominate even when formal approaches are called for?[56]

What is to guarantee that the right pattern or illness script will be selected?[49] And what if the patterns or scripts stored in the individual knowledge base are in some way mistaken or faulty? Given that our intuition is not perfect and that rational analytic thought is too time consuming, when should we trust our clinical intuition and when is a more systematic rational approach needed?

A RCT does not generate universal and generalizable knowledge, but rather reports observations about treatment effects in populations of individuals who share some qualities but not others, under certain specific circumstances.[21] The clinician must decide whether the patient-at-hand resembles the 'average' patient provided by the research closely enough to warrant incorporating the conclusion of that research into that patient's care. How closely the patient-at-hand resembles the 'average' patient in a study will determine how much weight should be given to the results.[21] When evaluating a health-care intervention, one would always like to be able to review the results of more than one study.[36] Direct evidence is preferred, because it does not require any assumptions about the integrity of the links needed to connect the different bodies of evidence.[36] Many, if not most, EB clinical practice guidelines are based on indirect evidence because they rely on a chain of evidence.[36]

How should we weigh all components of an EBM integrated approach to clinical decision-making correctly? Knowledge on the effectiveness of treatments remains contextual knowledge, which is strongly dependent on presuppositions about what questions are important, what sort of connections are meaningful and how these should be clarified.

Medical uncertainty not only persists because clinicians and patients must act on imperfect information, but also because much medical knowledge functions tacitly.[40]

If we now – by using EBM – supposedly better understand how to critically appraise evidence, we should have an equally structured and organized method for how to use the best evidence in conjunction with physician clinical expertise (knowledge, attitude, skills), health-care setting, patient expectations, values, preferences and choices.[10] Now we just need someone to tell us how to perform this integration of research into clinical work in clear operational terms, according to which criteria and in which explicit steps.[10] Alas, no such method exists.

So far, we do not have a clear guide to help make such a desirable integration work.

The strategies reviewed are neither proof against error nor always consistent with statistical rules of inference. Errors that can occur: failure to generate the correct hypothesis, misperception or misreading the evidence, misinterpretations of the evidence.[58] Restructuring and reformulating should occur as data are being obtained and the clinical picture evolves.[58] Often, we are updating opinion with imperfect information.

18. Not everything can, must, or will be studied

Five million years of evolution and fifty years of research have shown that mother's milk is good for babies.

Far from all clinical situations have been tested by randomized, controlled, double-blind, adequately powered studies. And indeed, it is only in utopia that a situation will exist wherein all medical decision-making will be based only upon trials; as Cochrane wrote: "We will never get sufficient medical personnel of the right calibre for this sort of work."[28] Indeed, a thorough literature search for every single medical encounter is beyond the reality of daily practice.

If no great doubt exists, we might better focus on real scientific dilemmas and clinically relevant questions that need to be taken care of, than spending a lot of time and research money on finding answers we already know. Clinical investigators occupied with the search-and-aggregate mission of meta-analysis are diverted from doing other useful research.[3] As the EBMWG stated: the problem selected for critical appraisal must be one that the learners recognize as important, feel uncertain about, and do not fully trust expert opinion on; in other words, they must feel it is worth the effort to find out what the literature says on a topic.[19] It cannot indeed be required that everything should be proved, since that is impossible; but one can see to it that all propositions which are used without being proved, are expressly stated as such, so that it is clearly known on what the whole structure rests.[9]

For some questions, appropriate trials would be difficult to design or unethical to carry out. For some, one might ask: who would volunteer? RCT results will be available for only a limited scope of therapeutic options.[3] The rest of these topics are likely to be altered by tomorrow's experience.[58]

Because many medical practices have not been rigorously evaluated, we do not know, what their impact on effectiveness and safety are. More than half of all medical treatments, and perhaps as many as 85% surgical treatments have not been tested in trials.[36]

The OM, however, exaggerated its usefulness by understating several difficulties. For instance, at a purely practical level, what commitment of time and money will be required to determine the effectiveness of the many commonly used-and continuously evolving-medical procedures?

Feyerabend already warned against 'tyranny of method'; in his opinion following strict methodological rules would have been and will be catastrophic – some important scientific advances never would have occurred.[37] We need to remember that many of the best treatment options available were never proven in a trial.

Giant steps were hardly made anymore during the last decades; as Charlton noted a general deceleration of innovation exists since the 1960s. Widely popularized hierarchical rules of EBM have resulted in the stifling of scientific debate and have threatened scientific progress.

19. Only looking at RCTs will not work

The scope of randomized trials is limited by direct applicability only to 'average' patients, by the absence of RCTs for prophylactic therapy of 'risk factors', by 'grey zones' that have not been clarified by RCTs, by pathophysiologic principles for which RCTs would be inappropriate or unethical, and by the many clinical decisions for which RCTs are not possible or pertinent.[3]

Regarding tests of significance, Hill already stated that "There are numerous situations in which they are totally unnecessary – because the difference is grotesquely obvious, because it is negligible, or because, whether it be formally significant or not, it is too small to be of any practical importance. What is worse the glitter of the *t* table diverts attention from the inadequacies of the fare."[59]

Objective evidence for effective therapy is of two kinds. The first is the 'miracle cure', when effectiveness is not in doubt among rational and informed parties. These are treatments which improve a predictably bad prognosis: a previously fatal disease is no longer fatal, a drug has a quick and dependably curative effect in all patients, surgery restores anatomical normality etc.[60] Described by Cochrane as: "The drugs whose effect on immediate mortality were so obvious that no trials were necessary" or "therapies with no backing from RCTs, which are justified by their immediate and obvious effect."[28] Chalmers, Sackett and Silagy wrote: "when care has such striking effects, (...) carefully controlled research is seldom necessary to identify whether the prescriptions and proscriptions of doctors and other health professionals are more likely to do good than harm."[61]

The second kind of objective evidence is necessary when prognosis is unpredictable, and a group of patients must be studied under scientific conditions. The upshot is the double-blind RCT, which is a technique for quantifying natural remissions and the placebo effect in order to differentiate them from specific treatment. We need to realize that randomized trials are necessary if we doubt whether the one treatment is better than the other. So, if there is no knowledge to prove otherwise. If for example a pharmaceutical company makes a claim that the new drug is superior to the existing ones, it is necessary to show the evidence in a RCT.

Average results for efficacy have been highly successful in letting policy makers and pharmaceutical manufacturers make such decisions as whether streptomycin is beneficial enough to warrant industrial production, or whether bypass surgery is worth its risks and costs in patient with coronary disease.[3]

Clinicians frequently encounter situations in which there is no relevant evidence from either basic or applied research. Until many of the gaps are closed clinical experience and reasoning (based on principles derived from basic scientific research) must be applied to traverse the many gray zones of practice. Even when evidence exists, difficulties arise when it is inconclusive, inconsistent with previous studies, irrelevant to clinical realities or of poor quality. And last but not least, in few research studies are the results reported in the context of the totality of available evidence.

RCTs can be helpful for determining whether an intervention will reliably produce the desired effect under well-controlled, essentially ideal circumstances. On the other hand, RCTs may not tell us much about how effective treatments are when they are used in everyday practice by ordinary clinicians and patients.[4] To quote Hill again: "The sample may be akin to that of the man who had a mind to sell his house and carried a piece of brick in his pocket, which he showed as a pattern to encourage purchasers."[59] The RCT may be a powerful tool but it is not a gold standard, and needs to be interpreted with a similar degree of skepticism as results from 'lower' study designs.[62]

It was also stated that in the absence of systematic observation one must be cautious in the interpretation of information derived from clinical experience and intuition, for it may at times be misleading. I do agree with that, however, this is a two-way street; a single trial by a single institution may be as misleading as clinical experience. We must keep in mind that a fair ten times coin toss may also end up 8:2 for the different sides. Likewise, a single RCT can have an outcome that is further from the 'truth' than we usually think it is, because even a randomized factor might be unequally distributed. A small p-value may arise because the null hypothesis is false. But it can also mean that some mathematical aspect of the model was not correctly specified, that sampling was not a hundred percent random, that we accidentally switched the names of some factor levels, that we unintentionally, or intentionally, selected analyses that led to a small p-value, that we did not measure what we think we measured, or that a cable in our measuring device was loose.[63]

A treating physician must always draw inferences from the aggregate measures to his individual patient, so the evidence in EBM is necessarily at a remove from actual practice.[16] In fact, randomization, which EBM requires in evidence of therapeutic effectiveness, is a statistical method intended to wash out individuality – to render inconsequential any individual difference not specified in the research design.[16] EMB relies on probabilistic studies. RCTs measure average effects and do not necessarily match the local and complex situation of the individual patient.[17]

The 'average' patient, of course, does not exist.[44] Even patients with presumably identical disease processes present with variable histories and different examination results, at various stages of severity, with different values and priorities, as well as disparate emotional responses and psychological manifestations.[44] Modern clinical research seeks to avoid these potential confounders in assessing the efficacy of a particular intervention through the use of randomly selected control groups.[44] Important but usually omitted soft data are the types of symptoms, severity of symptoms, auxometry of illness and severity of the comorbidity.[3] A good clinician constantly uses this soft information for diverse clinical decisions. Intention-to-treat policy ignores all the events that happen after randomization, the additional therapeutic decisions and interventions evoked by those events, and the subsequent consequences.[3] The statistical technique of randomization obscures all aspects of individual variability even those that may be clinically relevant.[40] Non-quantifiable differences between individuals cannot be studied through the techniques of modern clinical research and, therefore cannot be incorporated into the evidence-based framework.[40]

The primary goal of clinical medicine, the benefit of the individual patient, is not directly addressed by the techniques of clinical research. The
results of empirical research cannot be applied to a particular individual
without the consideration of particular values, both of the professional
and the patient. Issues in personal preferences, psychosocial factors,
comfort and reassurance must be individualized and cannot suitably be
guided by published reports for an average patient.

20. Proper use

Clinical research continues to produce results which transferred to daily practice, will increasingly assist common sense. EBM has brought much needed thoroughness to assessing the achievements of modern medicine.[33]

More and better focus on epidemiology and statistics as well as ameliorating literature assessment did have positive impact on medical care. The quality of published papers in all journals has improved immensely and probably it will continue to do so. And I do concur with the necessity to ameliorate the quality of research and publications, and the importance of training clinicians to appraise research critically. In its original spirit, EBM succeeded in liberating us from authority as the only crucial indicator of what to learn, believe and do.[10]

Furthermore, many articles have been published instructing clinicians on how to access, evaluate, and interpret the medical literature. Proposals to apply the principles of clinical epidemiology to day-to-day practice have been put forward. An appeal to the best evidence has taught us to seek and find independently of others the evidence that gives us our understanding of health problems and directions for decision making.[10]

We have improved our ways of formulating appropriate questions and to clearly state problems to be solved as vital triggers for the entire EBM process.[10] We know how to retrieve relevant information for medical decisions and understanding from the increasingly voluminous maze of information available through various electronic and printed sources.[10]

Early guidelines tended to be strongly influenced by expert opinion. During the past decades, methods for identification, critical appraisal and syntheses of published evidence have become more formal, rigorous, quantitative, and sophisticated.

Important components of the GRADE approach are the recognition of how RCTs can be degraded as evidence; an acceptance that observational studies can provide strong evidence; an enhanced recognition of heterogeneity of perspectives regarding the interpretation of evidence; and pragmatic emphasis on flexibility in interpreting outcome measures.[6] These are all welcome developments that expand the range of application of EBM considerably and likely reflect an unacknowledged response to previous criticisms.[6]

In medical education, EBM teaches critical thinking and the value of scientific skepticism.[37] It allows clinicians to provide patients with information that can promote shared decision making.[39]

Because of the rapid growth of medical knowledge and the widening application of technology to medicine, there is a particular need for a continuing authoritative review of standards for both preventive and therapeutic strategies.[59]

Properly understood and applied, with its limits well delineated, epidemiological EB approaches can improve the *rigueur* of medical practice.[39]

21. Misuse

The consequence of standardizing both the patient and the moral considerations of how to manage him or her means that (a) patients who come in all shapes and sizes and with a vast range of co-morbidities, sociocultural influences, and personal idiosyncrasies – are wrongly assumed to conform to the 'ideal type' patient around which a trial was designed and b) the clinician is placed under powerful but clandestine moral pressure to align the management of this patient with the management of the ideal type.[49]

A barrier to EBM according to the EBMWG is: "People like quick and easy answers. Cookbook medicine has its appeal. Critical appraisal involves additional time and effort and may be perceived as inefficient and distracting from the real goal."[19] I fear that the opposite is true as much, the younger generation trained especially in the radicalized version of EBM, only searches in a guideline or systematic review to find the quick answer. They cannot help but practice 'cookbook' medicine, for they will have been provided none of the insight or skills that would enable them to successfully deviate from the 'recipe'.[39]

Important single studies, particularly other than RCTs may be omitted from the authorized collection.[3] The authoritative aura given to the collection, however may lead to major abuses that produce inappropriate guidelines or doctrinaire dogmas for clinical practice.[3]

While skills in the critical appraisal of reports of clinical research will remain vital to doctor education, medical training must directly address the limitations of relying primarily on empirical evidence for clinical decision making.

Following the tradition of EBM, medical doctors and researchers are increasingly trained in biostatistics and medical epidemiology, this has led to an explosion of expertise in study design and interpretation in spite of shrinking knowledge on pathophysiological principles.[31]

The existence of many thousands of EB-guidelines is no guarantee that the right section of the right guideline will be applied to the right patient at the right time.[49] On the contrary, the accumulation of unmanageable numbers of lengthy guidelines makes it ever more likely that the clinician at the front line will manage his or her patients using early categorization, frugal heuristics, and a privileging of operational rationality over case-based moral reasoning.[49] Experience as a patient suggests that I now receive far less attention from clinicians, whose primary focus now tends to be assigning their patients to a particular guideline.[49]

A critical interrogating attitude as opposed to a mechanical use of guideline recommendations or any other data is of great importance.[17] One must put emphasis on the importance of self-conscious questioning. As critical thinkers, we want to analyze and appraise whether or not the best evidence is correctly applied in argumentations about health problems under consideration.[64] Even the best evidence may be misused in flawed arguments. We need appraisal of evidence itself and appraisal of how such already critically appraised evidence is applied in argumentation in research and practice with understanding and decision making in mind.[64] Moreover, recommendations must be regarded as minimal standards, and it would be a serious error if health insurance agencies, ever considered them to be the maximal standards instead.[65]

The roots of EBM are in sociological terms a result of a challenge to physicians' authority – especially that of senior medics. The important question is whether such a challenge and analysis result in an improvement to things, and the answer depends on the relative legitimacy of 'traditional' physicians' authority compared with that of the practitioners of EBM.[26] It is, I would argue, seriously misleading to portray medical practice as distinctively based on arbitrary but socially sanctioned authority.[26] Charismatic expertise based upon subjective self-confidence unsupported by objective ability obviously occurs in medicine, but this is not distinctive to medicine.[26] Undermining of professional authority by EBM is made to seem un-controversially 'a good thing'; being a replacement of the arbitrary and subjective by the rigorous and objective.[26] But much of doctors' authority is perfectly reasonable; being based upon knowledge, understanding, training and experience; freely deferred to by patients who lack any of the pre-requisites.[26] Often enough, clinical authority is earned and appropriate, and to challenge such authority may be to replace it with something worse, and hence to be destructive of good practice.[26]

It is not a very pleasant matter to bring up the subject of doctor envy, but considering the barrage of criticism and misinterpretation which advocates of EBM have directed at doctors – accusing them of unreasoning inertia, innate conservatism, enslavement to commercial propaganda, blind prejudice and entrenched authoritarian attitudes – it might be reasonable at least to raise the matter.[26] It has become glaringly obvious that doctor envy and anti-medical prejudice are endemic throughout the paramedical domain.[26] Doctors enjoy a generally high status in the wider culture. Doctors have well-paid and secure jobs, dominant personalities, and a relatively unreflective yet rapidly decisive behavioral style that often leads to doctrinal clashes.[26]

The significance of anti-medical feeling can be seen in the barely disguised delight evinced by the paramedical and public health advocates of EBM when they contemplate the come-uppance which their approach will deliver to the medical profession. Following a good dose of EBM, medicine will (they hope) be wrested from the clutches of the paternalistic authoritarians and become the domain of information technologists, statisticians (and managers) operating a well-organized bureaucratic system on objective, explicit lines – and good riddance to the doctors![26] But before destroying what we have, it is worth asking whether the above rationalist utopia has any chance of delivering the goods. And in this we can be clear: the vison of practice put forward by EBM is untried, untested, incoherent and utopian.[26]

EBM as a system of health care is based upon a misreading of medical history, a misunderstanding of clinical science and a misinterpretation of epidemiology. At least the present 'system' of professional self-regulation works – how imperfectly.[26] And, furthermore, there is generally a high degree of public satisfaction limited mainly by the fact that the public do not have easier access to more of the same, rather than by their desire to have something utterly different along the lines of EBM.[26] Reform rather than revolution, is indicated. Traditional managerial and audit methods require a conveniently measurable output, and clinical services are notoriously difficult to quantify. However, quality-assurance audit concentrates not on performance but on the system – quality is defined and measured in terms of the operations of a control and feedback system. The 'evidence-based' movement in the health service provides exactly such a quality assurance system. As the 'implementation' moves on from evidence-based medicine, through evidence-based education, research and development, nursing, public health and health policy, we are witnessing the creation of an interlocking system to comprise an 'evidence-based' health service.[5] This would incorporate all aspects of health service practice, and be based-upon a process of standardized monitoring and interpretation of information. And since the only aspect of quality assurance not open to challenge is the legitimacy of the quality assurance system itself, EBM would permanently be insulated from criticism.[5]

However, the immaturity of EBM and its bias towards a narrow scientism pose considerable risks to the future viability and relevance of the entire initiative. We are engaged in a science-based rationalization of health care, as an alternative to arbitrary rationing. The new scientism in health services research and, by extension, health policy makes a spurious claim to provide certainty in a world of clinical uncertainty.[25] The dilemma facing policy makers, managers and practitioners, as well as the public in general, is that in most cases we are not dealing with a clearcut question of whether treatment is effective or ineffective. Rather, the questions are how effective, and to what degree of probability.[25]

What might protagonists of EBM have in mind? I think that they, mistakenly, call for a new type of authoritarianism, hidden behind an amorphous entity called EBM.[13] They suggest replacing healthy scientific debates, in which no one should claim authority over the truth, with authorities of scientific knowledge – readers of the literature who will announce a verdict about the evidence and ensure that their verdict is properly executed.[13] What is this entity that can decide on right and wrong in daily medical practice? Who claim that what they call evidence is more valid than another doctor's interpretation of empirical experience?

Overweening and unjustifiable ambition should be opposed, just as we ought to oppose the imposition of any system of rationalistic dictatorship based upon simplistic and incomplete analysis.[26] I see EBM, in its present form, as a dangerous delusion; erroneous in both rationale and conclusions, and a potentially lethal weapon in the hands of misguided regulators and reformers.[26]

22. How it should be?

According to the original *JAMA* paper, the former paradigm was based on different assumptions. However, this paper was a very simplified representation and an assumption in itself. Furthermore, it was written as if the assumptions from the former paradigm would be sufficient on their own, which I agree they are not. However, the evidence derived from these pillars might build strong cases. In the next step, that evidential level could have been raised with the additional incorporation of an epidemiological stone in the evidence pillar that consists of appropriate assessment of literature.

The effort to determine the outcomes and effectiveness of different medical interventions and to use that information as an aid to clinical decision-making is, I believe, a useful extension of basic clinical research.[4]

EBM also involves applying traditional skills of medical training. A sound understanding of pathophysiology is necessary to interpret and apply the results of clinical research. Understanding the underlying pathophysiology allows the clinician to better judge whether the results are applicable to the patient at hand and also has a crucial role as a conceptual and memory aid. Clinical judgement, with its use of personal experience, analogy and extrapolation, is still necessary in a system of EBM. Each step of the EBM process requires 'interpretive judgements'; many of these judgements necessary for the formulation of clinical practice guidelines will best be made by those with clinical expertise. Scientific evidence must be blended with a physician's experience, reasoning, and the knowledge of his or her patients and their preferences.

Expert opinion must not be devalued as unnecessary in a developed EBM, but seen as integral to the multifaceted medical knowledge that forms a better basis for patient care than the findings of even the most rigorous clinical research.[18,39] Empirical evidence, despite claims to the contrary, remains contextual knowledge, and expert opinion provides a vital contribution in defining the proper context of clinical research.[39] Evidence-based practice guidelines may in fact be viewed alternatively as examples of well-referenced expert opinion.

Effective clinical education requires both explicit instruction in and tacit demonstration of medical skills and judgement. The traditional apprenticeship model of medical education provides this kind of tacit learning through continual practice and observation by maximizing face-to-face interactions at the bedside.[40] Our good will, sincerity and energy and the years we invested in this domain deserve to be channeled in the best direction possible for the full benefit of patients and the community. With cornerstones including that clinical decisions should be based on all available evidence and that the clinical problem should determine the type of evidence to be sought.

Personal judgement is not a form of 'low-grade evidence' but the activity and rational obligation of each responsible individual, who attempts to balance all the different concerns and demands, to evaluate competing claims and 'warrants' for decisions in the diverse and often unique situations she or he faces.[43]

By unpacking the interpretation involved in integrating the knowledge sources, we might be able to perform this process more systematically and adequately. That can make the decisions more transparent.

The focus of attention will be less on the elimination of bias and more on understanding what a well-reasoned and well-justified decision can be.[35]

To rate the strength of evidence that emerges from a group of studies, one has to not only identify all relevant studies and to evaluate the quality of each individual study, but also assess the consistency of study results and the heterogeneity of key elements of study design to determine the comparability of studies.[36] Key considerations when evaluating a body of evidence include whether the approach used to identify potentially pertinent literature was comprehensive and unbiased, and whether bias was avoided in evaluating, synthesizing, and interpreting available evidence.[36] Approaches for rating the strength of a body of evidence also have become richer, based on considerations of the quality (internal validity of each study), quantity (for example, the number of studies or aggregate sample size), consistency (the extent to which similar findings are reported in studies that employed similar or different study designs), and coherence of evidence (do the findings make sense as a whole?).[36] Even so, a synthesis of the results of multiple studies often involves not only quantitative analysis but also substantial subjectivity in the form of judgements regarding the admissibility (that is, is a particular study fatally flawed, and hence to be ignored), relevance, or importance of individual pieces of evidence.[36] That factors aside from strength of evidence are determinative in decision making indicates that such factors require a justification that EBM cannot supply.[6]

EBM has embraced the view that 'rational thinkers' respect their evidence and that a wise man proportions his belief to the evidence.[37] Indeed one should! Understanding of medical epistemology can provide for an explicit defense of a more 'common sense' practice of medicine that has been called for time and time again. Beyond EBM there lies a whole world of good practice and real evidence which has been largely forgotten or obfuscated by rhetoric.[5] Alternative, more effective models of health service organization are available – including self-regulating professionals embedded in a facilitating administrative structure; while superior modes of clinical investigation would emphasize rigorous clinical science, close observation of practice including individual case studies, whole population studies and representative population sampling – with mega/meta-population epidemiology again relegated to its proper, subordinate, role of precise measurement.[5] We need an approach to medical epistemology that places the concept of judgement at the center, and treats the project of how to cultivate good judgement as its central concern.[43]

The emphasis of EBM on skepticism and uncertainty – we will never be sure of the magnitude of the effects of our treatments or the power of our diagnostic tests – is central to the approach and agrees with the philosophical view that scientific knowledge is never complete and ultimately fallible.[37] However, a balance is necessary between the use of guidelines based on what is known to be effective to encourage improved practice on the one hand and the retention by the medical profession of the capacity to apply clinical judgement on the other.[25] The goal of a search for evidence may not be the truth per se, but finding enough information to reasonably support a decision. I am convinced that evidence-based medicine can only keep that name, if it intends to use all evidence. It should be aimed at trying to prove an assertion to the best of our knowledge and possibilities. Attempting assessment before all available evidence is obtained and considered in its entirety is a mistake implicit in a posited hierarchy equating real world evidential reliability with theoretical reliability of methods used to obtain evidence: a logical non-sequitur.[7]

We must be heading towards the development of an adequate epistemology of medical practice that retains EBM's valuable insights without its faulty precepts.[40] Cochrane himself once wrote: "One should be delightfully surprised when any treatment at all is effective, and always assume that a treatment is ineffective unless there is evidence to the contrary."[28] But still adhering to such orthodoxy, taking it all literally, hurts too much.[66] That's why I like to end with Cochrane's wise words that might concur with the main motive of this booklet: "It is, I suppose, reasonable for clinicians not to be as obsessional as epidemiologists."[28]

Acknowledgments

The author likes to thank Erwin van der Veen, Thomas Muehlberger, Paul Hamberg, Sandra Tanenbaum, Elliot Shevel and Klaas van der Els for their willingness to read and comment on this booklet and/or on previous work, for their stimulating remarks, for good advice and healthy debates.

Previous articles by the author

De Ru JA, Van Benthem PP, Janssen LM. All evidence is equal, but some is more equal than others. Otol Neurotol 2010;31:551-3. http://dx.doi.org/10.1097/mao.0b013e3181cdda2a

De Ru JA, Van Benthem PPG. Malignant external otitis; changing faces. Int Adv Otol 2010;6:408-9

De Ru JA, Van Benthem PP. Combination therapy is preferable for patients with Ramsay Hunt Syndrome. Otol Neurotol 2011;32:852-855. http://dx.doi.org/10.1097/mao.0b013e31821a00e5

De Ru JA, De Groot JCMJ, Elshof JM. The review reviewed: stop publication bias. J Sci Explor 2012;3:635-646

De Ru JA, Van Benthem PPG, Van Wermeskerken GKA. Injudicious use of EBM: one step forward, two steps back. B-ENT 2014;10:245-249

De Ru JA. Septoplasty is a proven and effective procedure: an expert's view of a burning issue. B-ENT 2015;11:257-262

De Ru JA, Brennan PA, Martens E. Antiviral agents convey added benefit over steroids alone in Bell's palsy; decompression should be considered in patients who are not recovering. J Laryngol Otol 2015;129:300-6. http://dx.doi.org/10.1017/s0022215115000341

De Ru JA, Verdam FJ, Tabor MP, Van Wermeskerken GKA, Majoor MHJM. Commentary on Dutch guidelines regarding diseases of adenoids and tonsils. B-ENT 2017;13

De Ru JA, Koole A, Bol Raap RD, Teguh DN, Van Hulst RA. Hyperbaric oxygen for sudden sensorineural deafness: when guideline development goes astray. B-ENT 2017;13:97-104

Bayoumy AB, De Ru JA. Cochrane Systematic Review Antiviral Treatment for Bell's palsy; an opposing opinion! SN Comprehensive Clinical Medicine 2020; 2:928–932. http://dx.doi.org/10.1007/s42399-020-00339-4

Bayoumy AB, de Ru JA. Intramuscular Triamcinolon injection for severe hayfever. J Otol Rhinol 2020;9:1. http://dx.doi.org/10.37532/jor.2020.9(1).379

De Ru JA. Epidemiology, the cherry on the cake. Eur Arch Otorhinolaryngol 2022;279:1645-8

De Ru JA. Brutalized by bias. Ear, Nose & Throat Journal OnlineFirst, May 14, 2022 https://doi.org/10.1177/01455613221103084